The SHOCKING TRUTH About Palm Oil

How It Affects Your Health and the Environment

Dr. Bruce Fife

Piccadilly Books, Ltd.
Colorado Springs, CO

Every effort has been made to ensure that the information contained in this book is complete and accurate. However, neither the publisher nor the author is engaged in rendering professional advice or services to the individual reader. The information contained in this book is not intended as a substitute for consulting with your doctor.

Piccadilly Books, Ltd.
P.O. Box 25203
Colorado Springs, CO 80936, USA
info@piccadillybooks.com
www.piccadillybooks.com

Library of Congress Cataloging-in-Publication Data

Names: Fife, Bruce, 1952- author.
Title: The shocking truth about palm oil : how it affects your health and the environment / by Dr. Bruce Fife.
Description: Colorado Springs, CO : Piccadilly Books, Ltd., [2016] | Includes
   bibliographical references and index.
Identifiers: LCCN 2016010053 | ISBN 9780941599993 (trade pbk.)
Subjects: LCSH: Palm oil--Health aspects--Popular works. | Palm
   oil--Environmental aspects--Popular works.
Classification: LCC QP752.T63 F55 2016 | DDC 613.2/84--dc23 LC
record available at http://lccn.loc.gov/2016010053

Published in the USA

Contents

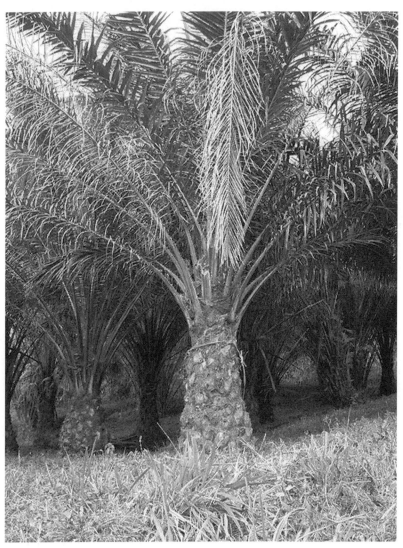

The oil palm *Elaeis guineensis*.

Chapter 1

The Benefits of Palm Oil May Surprise You

Over the past several years food manufacturers have been replacing hydrogenated vegetable oils in their products with a new, healthier oil. This product isn't really new. It's been in use for at least 5,000 years, but until recently it hasn't received much attention.

If you grab a package of Newman's Own chocolate chip cookies or examine the ingredients of Kellogg's Cracklin' Oat Bran cereal or read the ingredient label of any of dozens of food items in your local grocery or health food store you will find palm oil or palm fruit oil in place of the partially hydrogenated soybean or cottonseed oils that used to be there. You can even buy an entire bottle of it to use for cooking at home. What is this product? Why is palm oil being used in so many health foods and conventional foods now? Isn't palm oil a saturated fat? Why are manufacturers using this particular oil, aren't there better choices?

With the introduction of laws requiring the labeling of trans fats on food labels and the announcement by the United States Institute of Medicine stating that no level of trans fats are safe in the diet, food manufactures have been replacing hydrogenated vegetable oils—the primary source of trans fatty acids in our foods—with other oils, primarily with palm oil. Palm oil provides an excellent alternative to hydrogenated oils. Palm oil is highly resistant to oxidation and rancidity and can withstand the high temperatures used in cooking, baking, and deep frying. And, it is extraordinarily healthful, more so than most any other dietary oil.

In the past, palm oil was shunned by food manufacturers because of its high saturated fat content. Palm oil is composed of 50 percent saturated fat, 40 percent monounsaturated fat, and 10 percent polyunsaturated fat. Until recently, food manufacturers sensitive to customer fears of saturated fat have ignored palm oil in favor of hydrogenated vegetable oils. Now that hydrogenated vegetable oils have been linked to dozens of health problems, including heart disease and diabetes, customers are demanding a healthier choice.

Palm oil provides not just an alternative but a *healthy* alternative to hydrogenated and polyunsaturated fats in food preparation. Unlike hydrogenated vegetable oils, palm oil contains no toxic trans fatty acids. Like other vegetable oils it is completely cholesterol-free. Unlike polyunsaturated oils, such as corn or soybean oils, palm oil is not easily oxidized and does not produce toxic byproducts when heated. Palm oil is more stable than monounsaturated oils such as olive and canola oils with a smoke point of 437 degrees F (225 degrees C), making it ideal for use in commercial and home food preparation.

Some people question the use of palm oil as a replacement for hydrogenated oils, expressing a fear of saturated fat. That fear, however, is ungrounded. After more than three decades of intense study, palm oil has proven to be not only harmless but of great benefit in reducing risk of heart disease and improving overall health.

Studies conducted at the Universities of Louisiana and Wisconsin, the University of Reading in the UK, and the University of Western Ontario in Canada, have identified the following health benefits of palm oil:

• Reduces plaque in arteries, thus protecting against atherosclerosis and heart disease;

• Reduces blood cholesterol and improves the cholesterol ratio;

• Reduces blood clotting and keeps blood vessels dilated, thus reducing blood pressure and risk of heart attacks and strokes;

• Blocks the growth of cancer cells, especially in breast tissue;

• Enhances the efficiency of anti-cancer medications, such as Tamoxifen, by 45 percent.

Palm oil comes from the fruit of the oil palm (*Elaeis guineensis*). The oil palm originated in tropical Africa but is now also cultivated in Southeast Asia and South America. Palm oil has been a part of the human diet for thousands of

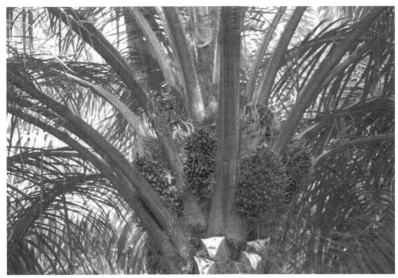

The oil palm produces fruit year round.

years. In the wild, animals regularly feast upon the fruit for its nutrient rich oil.

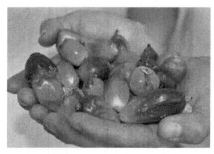

Palm fruit.

Palm fruit is about the size of a small plum and grows in large bunches. Each bunch may contain up to a 1000 individual fruits. The oil palm produces fruit continuously year round with a new bunch ripening about every month. So the fruit is always in season.

The oil is extracted from the fruit or pulp surrounding the seed. Palm fruit is a dark red color and produces an orange-red colored oil. This crude or virgin oil is called *red palm oil*. Red palm oil has undergone minimal processing, and therefore, retains most of the naturally occurring fat-soluble vitamins and other nutrients. The red color comes from beta-carotene and other carotenes. Red palm oil is the richest dietary source of beta-carotene, a precursor to vitamin A. For this reason, it is used as a means to fight vitamin A deficiency in children in many parts of the world.

Red palm oil is also the richest natural source of vitamin E. Palm oil contains two types of vitamin E—to-

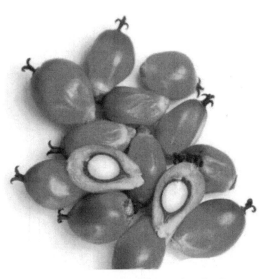

Palm oil is extracted from the fleshy pulp surrounding the kernel.

copherol and tocotrienol. Both types contain four subtypes—alpha, beta, gamma, and delta. The form of vitamin E we are most familiar with and the type commonly used in vitamin supplements is alpha-tocopherol. For many years alpha-tocopherol was believed to be the most biologically active form of vitamin E. The tocotrienols in palm oil exhibit far greater power, with up to 60 times the antioxidant activity of ordinary vitamin E. In essence, it is a super potent form of vitamin E.

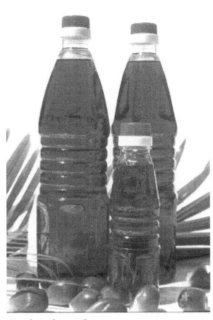

Red palm oil.

Red palm oil is loaded with a variety of other nutrients including CoQ10, lycopene, squalene, flavonoids, and phytosterols. With the high level of antioxidant carotenes, tocopherols, and tocotrienols, red palm oil is a superior dietary source for protective antioxidants. These nutrients have been shown to provide protection against a number of health conditions including premature aging, atherosclerosis, cancer, arthritis, diabetes, and Alzheimer's disease.

When red palm oil is processed into ordinary or "white" palm oil some of the nutrients are removed. Carotenes are affected most and nearly all of them are removed. However, most of the vitamin E and other nutrients remain, this still makes the oil a rich source of antioxidants and a very healthy cooking oil. White palm oil is the most common form used in commercial food processing. White palm oil is often sold in stores as trans fat-free vegetable shortening. Red palm oil is sold as a cooking oil.

Because of its distinctive orange-red color, red palm oil is easy to spot on store shelves. At room temperature it is semisolid, somewhat like soft butter. If refrigerated, it will harden. Out of the refrigerator, on a warm day, it will liquefy. You can use the oil when it is hard or soft. Nutritionally there is no difference. The oil is very stable and does not need to be refrigerated.

Red palm oil has a distinctive flavor and aroma. In cultures where palm oil is produced, it is an important ingredient in food preparation and gives the food much of its characteristic flavor. The oil has a pleasant, somewhat savory taste that enhances the natural flavor of meats and vegetables. The flavor complements soups, sauces, stir fries, eggs, and meats. In recipes that call for vegetable oil, butter, or margarine you can usually substitute red palm oil.

White palm oil is essentially tasteless. It is preferred where additional flavors are not wanted and is best for deep frying and baking. Palm oil is very heat stable and can be reused repeatedly for deep frying without creating off flavors or degrading the oil. Palm oil can be used to replace butter and shortening in baking and makes excellent pastries. In most recipes that call for butter or shortening you can use white palm oil instead. Of course, white palm oil can also be used in sautéing and frying just like red palm oil.

Red and white palm oils have a much higher nutritional profile than other cooking oils and contain a powerhouse of antioxidants. Unlike polyunsaturated oils, palm oil does not create harmful byproducts when heated, making it an ideal choice for home and commercial use. Next time you go to the market look for red palm oil or trans fat-free vegetable (palm) shortening.

Chapter 2

A Daily Dose of Vitamins
from A Cooking Oil

Palm oil, particularly virgin or red palm oil, is a traditional fat that has been a part of the human diet for thousands of years. For generations red palm oil has been revered as both a nutritious food and a valuable medicine. It was prized by the pharaohs of ancient Egypt as a sacred food. The oil was so highly valued that it was entombed with the pharaohs so that they would have access to it in the afterlife.

Throughout history palm oil has served as the primary source of dietary fat for countless numbers of people. Its nutritional and healing properties have been recognized for generations. Until modern medicine arrived, red palm oil was the remedy of choice for nearly every illness in many parts of Africa. When someone was sick, downing a cup full of palm oil was common. Even today many people in the villages rely on this age old method of treatment. Palm oil is regarded among many as essential in the diet for pregnant and nursing women in order to assure good health for the mother and child.

Today, medical doctors are recognizing the value of red palm oil in the treatment and prevention of malnutrition and vitamin deficiency diseases. Governments around the world are incorporating it into programs to wipe out deficiency diseases which are still rampant in many impoverished areas.

11

Carotenoids

Red palm oil not only supplies fatty acids essential for proper growth and development, but it is packed with an assortment of vitamins, antioxidants, and other phytonutrients important for good health. Red palm oil gets its name from its characteristic dark red color. The color comes from carotenoids such as beta-carotene and lycopene—the same nutrients that give tomatoes and carrots and other fruits and vegetables their rich red and orange colors.

Carotenoids are valuable nutrients and powerful antioxidants. They are also important because our body can convert them into vitamin A, an essential nutrient. Vitamin A deficiency can cause blindness, weaken bones, lower immunity, and adversely affect learning ability and mental function. Vitamin A is only found in animal foods. Such foods, are expensive and infrequently eaten by many impoverished people. Carotenoids in fruits and vegetables can supply the needed vitamin A if an adequate amount of fat is also consumed. Carotenoids require fat for conversion into vitamin A. Unfortunately, those who can't afford animal products often do not eat much fat either. Populations with ample carotenoid-rich foods available often suffer from vitamin A deficiency because they don't get enough fat in their diet.

Red palm oil provides a perfect solution. It supplies the needed fat and vitamin A precursors. Red palm oil is the richest dietary source of provitamin A carotenoids (beta-carotene and alpha-carotene). It has 15 times more provitamin A carotenoids than carrots and 300 times more than tomatoes. This has made it a valued resource in the treatment of vitamin A deficiency. Just one teaspoon a day of red palm oil supplies children with the daily recommend amount of vitamin A. Nursing mothers are encouraged to supplement their diet with palm oil to enrich their milk with the vitamin. Studies show that adding just a small amount of red palm oil into the diet can double or triple the amount of vitamin A in mother's milk.

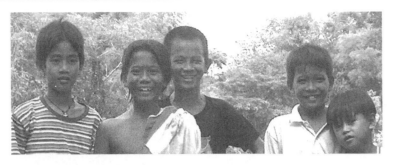

Saving Children's Lives

Red palm oil provides provitamin A carotenoids that can prevent and treat vitamin A deficiency—saving the sight and lives of millions of children worldwide.

It is estimated that 190 million preschool-age children worldwide suffer from vitamin A deficiency, with thousands of children going blind and dying each year as a result. Approximately 140 million more preschoolers suffer from subclinical vitamin A deficiency—that is, they consume enough vitamin A to prevent serious deficiency symptoms like corneal ulcers, but not enough for proper growth and development, or to prevent night blindness. Most of these children live in Asia and Sub-Saharan Africa.

Governments around the world are now instigating programs to include red palm oil in cookies, breads, and other baked goods to provide children who are suffering from vitamin A deficiency an inexpensive source for the vitamin. Nursing mothers can eat it to enhance the vitamin A content of their milk. Red palm oil solves one of the problems children and nursing mothers in poor areas of the world face. They may have access to carotenoid-rich vegetables, but they don't get enough fat in their diets to properly convert carotenoids into vitamin A. However, the provitamin A carotenoids in red palm oil come with their own source of oil, thus greatly enhancing carotenoid conversion and absorption. The oil palm is a native tree in many parts of Africa and is cultivated throughout Southeast Asia, so it provides an economically feasible and readily available dietary source of vitamin A that can solve the massive worldwide problem of vitamin A deficiency.

The children are not only getting the vitamin A they need, but other important nutrients as well. Red palm oil is a virtual powerhouse of nutrition. It contains by far, more nutrients than any other dietary oil. In addition to beta-carotene, alpha-carotene, and lycopene it contains at least 20 other carotenoids along with vitamin E, vitamin K, CoQ10, squalene, phytosterols, flavonoids, phenolic acids, and glycolipids. Palm oil is one of the richest natural sources of vitamin E. In addition to ordinary vitamin E, it also contains the highest amount of a super potent form of vitamin E known as tocotrienol.

Tocotrienols

There are two major types of vitamin E—tocopherol and tocotrienol—each consisting of four subtypes. The subtypes are identified by the prefix alpha, beta, gamma, and delta. The tocopherols (alpha-tocopherol, beta-tocopherol, gamma-tocopherol, and delta-tocopherol) are the most common. Alpha-tocopherol is the form of vitamin E we are most familiar with and the type commonly used in vitamin supplements and foods. When people talk about vitamin E they usually mean alpha-tocopherol. For many years alpha-tocopherol was believed to be the most biologically active form of vitamin E, and therefore, the most important. Recent studies now show that the other form of vitamin E, the tocotrienols, possess up to 60 times the antioxidant power of ordinary vitamin E and can have a much greater influence on health and disease prevention and treatment.

Tocopherols, the ordinary form of vitamin E, are relatively common in our diet. Tocotrienols, on the other hand, are harder to get. They are found in small amounts in some nuts, seeds, and grains. By far the most abundant source of these super antioxidants is in palm oil. Palm oil is one of the riches natural sources of vitamin E in general, and the richest source of tocotrienols.

Free radicals have been identified as the primary cause or a contributing factor in at least 60 common health problems

14

ranging from heart disease and cancer to arthritis and osteoporosis. Antioxidants quench the destructive action of free radicals. Because of its high antioxidant content, red palm oil has the potential to help prevent and even reverse many of these conditions. Therefore, palm oil may be of great benefit in helping to curb the onset and progression of many common health problems.

Heart disease is characterized by atherosclerosis or the buildup of plaque in the arteries. A number of studies have demonstrated the ability of antioxidants to prevent cholesterol oxidation and, thereby, arrest the development of atherosclerosis. Although ordinary vitamin E is a potent antioxidant it has only shown modest benefit in this respect. Palm tocotrienols, however, have shown to very effective in stopping and reversing atherosclerosis, and therefore, protecting against heart attacks and strokes.

Cardiovascular Health

Over the past three decades researchers have painstakingly studied palm oil's effect on cardiovascular health. The results have been surprising to researchers. Although high in saturated fat, it appears to protect against heart disease.

Studies show that adding palm oil into the diet can remove plaque buildup in arteries and therefore, reverse the process of atherosclerosis. This has been demonstrated in both animal and human studies. In one study, for instance, 50 subjects were divided into two equal groups. All the participants had been diagnosed with atherosclerosis and had suffered at least one stroke. At the beginning of the study the degree of blockage of their carotid arteries ranged from 15 to 79 percent. Without any other changes to their diets or medications, half of the subjects began taking a daily palm oil supplement. The other half received placebos and served as the control. The degree of atherosclerosis was monitored using ultrasound scans over an 18 month period. In the group receiving palm oil, atherosclerosis was halted in 23 of the 25 subjects. In seven

15

of these subjects atherosclerosis was not only stopped but regressed. In comparison, none of those in the control group showed any improvement, in fact, the condition in 10 of them worsened.[1] This study demonstrated that palm oil can not only stop, but even reverse atherosclerosis.

Removing plaque is not the only way palm oil protects against strokes and heart attacks. Palm oil can also improve cholesterol values. In a study at the University of Illinois College of Medicine researchers demonstrated a 10 percent decrease in total cholesterol in 36 hypercholesterolemic (high cholesterol) subjects given palm oil capsules for four weeks. A follow-up study of 16 subjects resulted in a 13 percent lowering of total cholesterol.[2]

In another study 31 subjects took a palm oil supplement every day for 30 days. No other changes were made to their diets. They continued to eat whatever they desired. The results showed that palm oil supplementation lowered both total cholesterol and LDL (bad) cholesterol in all the volunteers. The magnitude of reduction of total cholesterol ranged from 5 to 35.9 percent and the reduction of LDL cholesterol ranged from 0.9 to 37 percent. What was even more important was the effect the palm oil had on the cholesterol ratio. The cholesterol ratio was reduced in 78 percent of the subjects, demonstrating a highly significant and favorable response to supplementation.[3]

Another type of LDL cholesterol is lipoprotein(a) or Lp(a). It is similar in structure to LDL but contains an adhesive protein that enhances its ability to stick to artery walls. Lp(a) has been identified as a separate and distinct risk factor for heart disease. In fact, Lp(a) is associated with ten times the risk of elevated LDL. Cholesterol-lowering drugs have been ineffective in lowering Lp(a) levels. Several studies have shown that tocotrienols are effective in reducing Lp(a) and thus reduce risk of heart disease.[4, 5]

Palm oil helps maintain proper blood pressure. This powerful antioxidant inhibits platelets from sticking to one another, thereby "thinning" the blood. The high antioxidant content of the oil quenches harmful free radicals, reduces inflammation, and assists in keeping blood vessels properly dilated so that circulation remains normal and blood pressure stays under control.

In one study researchers induced inflammation in the arteries of test animals. Inflammation causes swelling which narrows artery passageways, restricting blood flow to vital organs such as the heart. Half of the test animals received palm oil in their diet while the other half served as the control. In the control group artery passageways were severely constricted and 42 percent of the animals died. However, those that received the palm oil showed far less inflammation and constriction resulting in a 100 percent survival rate.

Tocotrienols also strengthen the heart so that it can better withstand stress. Researchers can purposely induce heart attacks in lab animals by cutting off blood flow to the heart. This causes severe injury and death. However, if the animals are fed palm oil the survival rate is greatly increased, injury is minimized, and recovery quicker.[6]

After looking at studies like this it becomes obvious that palm oil protects against heart disease. This is confirmed in populations where palm oil consumption is particularly high. Heart disease in Malaysia, Indonesia, Papua New Guinea, and Nigeria—where palm oil is a major source of visible fat in the daily diet—is among the lowest in the world.[7]

Cancer Prevention

The high antioxidant content of palm oil makes it a potent anticancer food. Palm tocotrienols are especially benefical in this respect. Antioxidants have long been known to offer protection against various forms of cancer. Tocotrienols being highly potent antioxidants have demonstrated remarkable anticancer properties far superior to most other antioxidants.

Studies show palm tocotrienols inhibit the growth of skin, stomach, pancreas, liver, lung, colon, prostate, breast and other cancers. Most of the research to date has been done with breast

17

cancer where tocotrienols show great promise. They not only prevent cancer from taking hold but actively block its growth and initiate apoptosis—a process where diseased cells commit suicide. This is a normal process that is programmed into all of our cells in order to remove old and diseased cells. However, in cancer cells this process is blocked and affected cells continue to multiply and grow without restraint. Ordinary vitamin E, does not induce programmed cell death in cancer cells. Only tocotrienols have this effect.

Initial research has been so impressive that cancer researchers have called tocotrienols the most powerful natural anticancer substances known to science.[8] That's quite a bold statement, but illustrates the potential tocotrienols have in cancer prevention and treatment.

Brain Disorders

One of the worst things that can happen to us as we age is to lose our mental capabilities. Fortunately for us, tocotrienols can come to our rescue.

Two of the most significant factors that affect brain function are oxidative stress and poor circulation. Oxidative stress generates free radicals that damage brain and nerve tissue. Poor circulation affects the brain by restricting oxygen and glucose which are vital for proper brain function. Researchers have found correlations between oxidative stress and reduced blood flow to the brain to senile dementia, Alzheimer's disease, Parkinson's disease, Huntington's disease, and even schizophrenia. All of these conditions involve brain cell death. Tocotrienols aid the brain by reducing oxidative stress and improving blood flow.

Researchers can mimic much of the destruction seen in the above neurological disorders by feeding test animals glutamate—an amino acid that in large amounts kills brain cells. Glutamate is used by researchers to induce neurological damage in lab studies. We get glutamate in our diet from monosodium glutamate (MSG), soy protein isolate, and hydrolyzed soy protein, which are commonly added to foods. The primary action of cell death is caused by free radicals. Ordinary vitamin E is not strong enough to prevent glutamate-induced cell death. But palm tocotrienols can quench the destructive action of glutamate. In laboratory studies tocotrienol-treated neurons maintain healthy growth and motility even in the presences of excess glutamate.[9]

Dietary Supplement

The combination of a full spectrum of vitamin E (tocopherols and tocotrienols), carotenes, and other antioxidants makes palm oil a super antioxidant food. Red palm oil is loaded with so many nutrients and antioxidants it's like a natural dietary supplement. In fact, it is currently being encapsulated and sold as a vitamin supplement.

Supplements made from real foods are far better than purified synthetic supplements. When you take an ordinary vitamin E supplement, you are only getting alpha-tocopherol—one of eight of the forms of vitamin E. All forms of vitamin E are important and have slightly different effects and benefits on our health. Alpha-tocopherol isn't even the most potent or effective form of vitamin E. The palm tocotrienols are much better.

One table-spoon of red palm oil supplies more than enough vitamin E to meet daily requirements for an adult. The advantage of getting vitamin E from a food rather than a

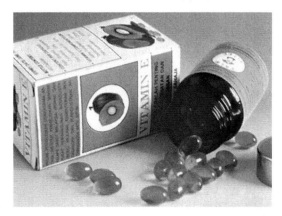

dietary supplement is that you get a full range of tocopherols and tocotrienols as well as many other naturally occurring nutrients that work synergistically together to improve health.

Palm oil is currently being used as a food ingredient and dietary supplement throughout the world to fight nutritional deficiencies and malnutrition. It is literally saving the lives of millions of children. It is a food and a nutritional supplement combined as one. In government programs for the treatment of nutritional deficiencies, palm oil is simply incorporated into the food. It's easy for a child to get a teaspoon of red palm oil when it is used to cook vegetables or bread.

The best way to take palm oil is to incorporate it into daily food preparation. Simply use it in place of other oils in recipes. Palm oil is an excellent choice for cooking and baking. The high saturated and monounsaturated fatty acid content (90 percent) makes palm oil a very heat resistant and stable oil. It has a high smoke point of 437 degrees F. The high saturated fat and antioxidant content makes it extremely resistant to oxidation and free-radical formation.

Research is showing that the antioxidant power of red palm oil can be of help in protecting against a variety of additional health problems including osteoporosis, asthma, cataract, macular degeneration, arthritis, and liver disease. It can even stunt the processes that promote premature aging. It's no wonder it was regarded as a sacred food by the ancient Egyptians. Red palm oil is not just for pharaohs, it's available to everyone. It is sold as a cooking oil and as a dietary supplement at most good health food stores and online. For more information about the health benefits of tocotrienols and palm oil I recommend my book *The Palm Oil Miracle*.

Chapter 3

A Healthy Alternative to Trans Fats or an Environmental Disaster?

A Better Choice

"No level of trans fats is safe," so says the United States Institute of Medicine. After an extensive three-year review of all published studies on the effects of trans fatty acids on human health, the Institute of Medicine made this announcement. The scientific evidence was clear, consumption of trans fatty acids found in hydrogenated vegetable oils increases the risk of coronary heart disease, diabetes, metabolic syndrome, and other health problems.

Trans fats (i.e., trans fatty acids) are created when vegetable oils are bombarded with hydrogen atoms in a process called hydrogenation. Hydrogenated vegetable oils have been popular in food processing because they harden liquid vegetable oil and make them more resist to oxidization and retard spoilage—necessary for packaged, prepared foods. Liquid vegetable oils are unsuitable because they oxidize easily, readily develop off flavors, and lack the firmness needed for baking. However, in the process of hydrogenating polyunsaturated vegetables oils, artificial fat molecules known as trans fatty acids, are created. These fatty acids are foreign to the human body and cause all manner of mischief.

Hydrogenation

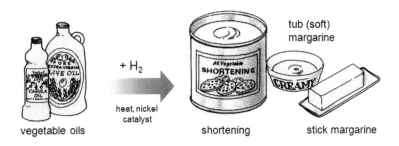

vegetable oils $+ H_2$ heat, nickel catalyst → shortening, tub (soft) margarine, stick margarine

Prior to the announcement by the Institute of Medicine, hydrogenated vegetable oils were found in most every packaged food on the grocery shelves and was used extensively in the food service industry. Ingredient labels listing partially hydrogenated vegetable oils, margarine, and shortening all contained unknown amounts of trans fats.

In response to the announcement, The Food and Drug Administration (FDA) mandated that food manufacturers must list the amount of trans fats in the Nutrition Facts panels on food labels. With the publicity surrounding the new labeling laws people have become more aware of the dangers of consuming trans fats. Fearing customers would hesitate to buy products knowing that they contained trans fats, food manufacturers began looking for suitable alternatives.

Food and cosmetic manufacturers cannot simply replace hydrogenated oils in their products with another type of vegetable oil. The characteristics of soy, corn, canola, safflower, sunflower, and other vegetable oils are not suitable for most food and cosmetic use. Most vegetable oils are too liquid and too fragile for commercial use. Using these types of oils would dramatically shorten shelf life of the products and cause some serious health concerns. The trouble with all

Nutrition Facts

Serving Size 1 Tbsp (14g)
Servings Per Container about 32

Amount Per Serving

Calories 100   Calories from Fat 100

	% Daily Value*
Total Fat 11g	**17%**
Saturated Fat 2.5g	**12%**
Trans Fat 2.5g	
Cholesterol 0mg	**0%**
Sodium 105mg	**4%**
Total Carbohydrate 0g	**0%**
Dietary Fiber 0g	0%
Sugars 0g	

INGREDIENTS: WHOLE GRAIN POPCORN, PARTIALLY HYDROGENATED SOYBEAN OIL, SALT, NATURAL AND ARTIFICIAL FLAVOR [MILK], COLOR ADDED, FRESHNESS PRESERVED BY PROPYL GALLATE.

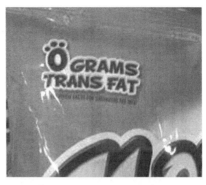

Labeling laws require food manufacturers to indicate the amount of tras fats in their products (left). Some companies (above) are taking advantage of consumers growing awareness of the dangers of trans fats and are boldly marking their products as containing 0 grams of trans fats.

these vegetable oils is that they are all highly polyunsaturated. Polyunsaturated fats break down, become oxidized and go rancid, very quickly. When subjected to heat, such as in cooking or in commercial processing, they degrade rapidly producing health-damaging free radicals. This has been a known problem with polyunsaturated oils and why you don't see them used more often in packaged foods.

In an effort to find a replacement for hydrogenated oils, food chemists have been busy fractionating fats and oils, creating new fats, and recombining them in various ways to create relatively hard fats that are trans fat-free and contain as little saturated fat as possible. Agricultural scientists are also experimenting with genetically modified plants to find a solution. Some of these manufactured oils are now being incorporated into our foods.

A far simpler and healthier solution is to go back to the fats we used before we had hydrogenated oils—traditional fats that have been used successfully for generations. Many food manufacturers are doing that. One traditional fat that is gaining wider use is palm oil. Compared to other fats, palm oil is far superior in nutrient content and cooking properties. Palm oil is highly resistant to oxidation and rancidity and can withstand the high temperatures used in cooking, baking, and deep frying. Palm oil is also less expensive than the contrived fats chemists have attempted to make to replace hydrogenated oils.

As hydrogenated vegetable oils are being removed, palm oil is becoming the oil of choice to take its place. When you look at ingredient labels and see "palm oil" listed, you know you are getting a healthy trans fat-free oil packed with nutrients.

Environmental Concerns

Because of the many advantages of palm oil, its acceptance and use has steadily grown as people have gained greater awareness of the dangers of consuming hydrogenated vegetable oils and with polyunsaturated vegetable oil in general. Prior to the trans fat labeling law, soybean oil was by far the most commonly used oil in the world. Since that time it has gradually lost its market share to palm oil. Today palm oil has taken over the number one spot and accounts for 31 percent of all vegetable oils traded internationally.

Palm oil is now a common ingredient in non-hydrogenated margarines, biscuits, breads, breakfast cereals, instant noodles, chocolates, ice creams, shampoos, lipsticks, candles, detergents, and other prepared foods and cosmetics. Hundreds of products that once contained hydrogenated soybean, cottonseed, and corn oils, now use palm oil.

Despite the replacement of health-damaging hydrogenated vegetable oils from most commercial products with the much healthier palm oil, not everyone has been so accepting

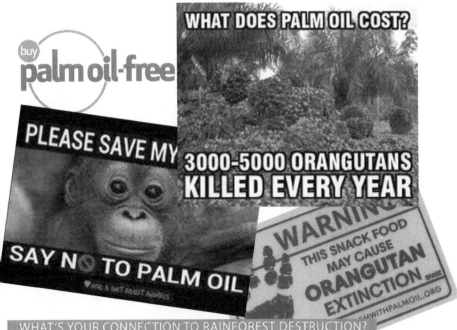

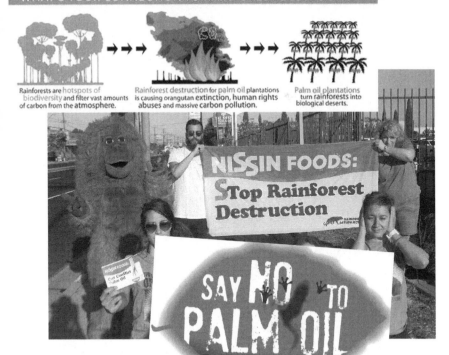

Critics claim that palm oil is harming the environment.

of the change. The palm oil industry has taken a beating in the international press, with accusations of deforestation, unsustainable farming practices, and damage to native wildlife habitats.

Critics claim that clearing land for oil palm plantations has led to widespread deforestation in Indonesia and Malaysia as well as other regions. This has pushed many species to the brink of extinction, such as rhinos, elephants, orangutans, and tigers. In some cases, forest clearance has forced indigenous peoples off their land, deprived them of their livelihood and reduced essential ecosystem services such as clean water and fertile soil. The destruction of tropical rainforests, they claim, is a major contributor to climate change, as felled and burned trees and vegetation release methane and other greenhouse gases into the atmosphere. Moreover, because fire is often used as a cheap and quick means to clear land for agriculture, the resulting air pollution can block out the sun and threaten human health both near and far.

Numerous green organizations have taken up the cause and have vigorously campaigned against the use of palm oil. Buying products that contain palm oil only supports the mass deforestation and the destruction of wildlife that is occurring they say. Nationwide boycotts have been called for to stop people from purchasing any product containing palm oil and encourage food and cosmetic manufacturers to replace palm oil with soy, corn, canola, sunflower, safflower, or other vegetable oils.

If these claims are true, it is certainly an issue to be concerned about. But what is the truth? Is the increasing use of palm oil destroying forests, wildlife, and the environment? In the following chapters, we will investigate the truth behind the palm oil scare and see who really is destroying forests and causing widespread damage to the planet.

Chapter 4

Genetically Engineered Foods

Are Genetically Engineered Foods the Wave of the Future?

The United States Food and Drug Administration (FDA) recently announced that it has approved the sale of genetically engineered (GE) salmon for human consumption, making it the first genetically altered animal to be cleared for sale in supermarkets and restaurants. The genetically altered salmon are engineered to produce a higher level of growth hormone, causing them to reach market size in just half the time as conventionally raised salmon.

More GE foods are on the way. Korean scientists have developed hogs with extraordinarily large backsides, the part that pork-eaters particularly value. These grotesque-looking hogs resemble something you might imagine from creepy offspring of animals exposed to high levels of radiation more than they do potential sources of food for human consumption. Their appearance is enough to turn anybody's stomach.

Developing animals that produce a greater percentage of prime cuts of meat is a major goal of genetic scientists. However, not all of the genetic manipulations are focused on producing larger animals or animals with grossly expanded body parts.

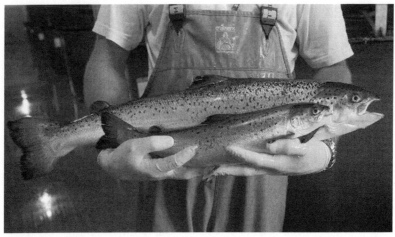

GE salmon have genes from a Chinook salmon and an ocean pout—a type of eel—that make more than the usual dose of growth hormone, so they reach market size in half the time as natural salmon. A genetically engineered salmon from AquaBounty Technologies, rear, with a conventionally raised sibling roughly the same age.

Some animals are developed to enhance or remove certain characteristics. Researchers in Minnesota are developing milk and beef cattle that have no horns. Ranchers typically de-horn cattle when they are calves to make them less likely to inure other animals or the people who handle them. One drawback so far with hornless dairy cows is that they don't produce any milk, just another glitch to be worked out with further genetic manipulations. In New Zealand scientists have engineered cows that produce milk without the proteins that trigger milk allergies; now everyone can enjoy GE milk.

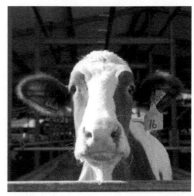

A genetically altered hornless cow.

Even insects are being genetically manipulated. Genetically altered mosquitoes will soon be released in the Florida Keys as an attempt to reduce the risk of dengue fever. There is no guarantee that this experiment will work. Introducing species of animals and insects from one part of the world into other

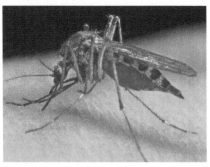

Scientists plan to release genetically engineered mosquitos into the wild.

areas to control pests has generally ended up as environmental disasters. A genetically altered insect is foreign to the entire world so there is no telling what might happen.

Farmers have been using GE crops since the 1990s. Currently as much as 80 percent of the foods in the typical American grocery store contain GE ingredients. Proponents of GE foods claim that they are the wave of the future and will increase crop yields and provide a means to feed a growing world population and thus end world hunger. A noble cause indeed, but is it true? Will converting conventional crops to GE varieties end world hunger? Will it even increase crop yields? Or, as some critics claim, will it be a colossal failure or even worse, usher in an environmental catastrophe and economic disaster?

We hear a lot about the potential harm caused by consuming gluten, sugar, artificial sweeteners, trans fats, preservatives, and such. Of all the ingredients in our foods, what ones are potentially the most troubling? While all of those mentioned have their issues, potentially the most troubling foods are those that contain GE or genetically modified (GM) ingredients. Not only do they pose a threat to our health, but they are dangerous to the environment. What makes them especially troubling is the fact that in places like the US, there are no labeling laws (as of this writing) to inform you which foods contain GE ingredients.

The biotech firms that produce GE seeds, the Grocery Manufacturers Association (a consortium of food producers and manufacturers) and their friends in government are continually telling us that GE foods are completely safe and there is no need to worry. Thus, causing many people to be in a state of ignorance about the real dangers of these foods.

Awareness about the potential risks of genetically engineered foods is growing. This is due largely because of the publicity generated by individual states that have put to vote whether or not to require foods that contain GE ingredients be identified on the label. Giant corporations and their associates like Monsanto (and other biotech companies) and the Grocery Manufacturers Association have been fighting bitterly to prevent consumers from knowing what's in their foods. The latest polls suggest more than 90 percent of Americans now want to know what's in their foods (according to a poll conducted by MSNBC).

A number of scientists have raised warnings about the danger of GE foods. The evidence is strong enough to convince many governments to ban them or at least establish labeling laws so their citizens know what they are buying. Currently 64 nations require the labeling of foods containing GE ingredients including Austria, Germany, Italy, New Zealand, Australia, Greece, Poland, Malaysia, Brazil, Russia, India, and even China.

Most Americans are totally unaware that they are already eating GE foods. There are no labeling laws at present to inform them. Since the 1990s GE foods have slowly and quietly filtered into our food system. Today, approximately 80 percent of the foods sold in stores and restaurants contain at least some GE ingredients.

About 90 percent of all corn, soybeans, rapeseed/canola, sugar beets, and cotton grown in the US are genetically altered.

If you eat anything that contains these foods you are most likely eating GE products. You say you don't eat corn or soy. Think again. Corn is in almost everything. Corn is used in corn meal and flour, oil, and high fructose corn syrup, also referred to as simply "corn syrup" on food labels. How many products are cooked in corn oil or contain high fructose corn syrup? Lots! Most foods now are sweetened with high fructose corn syrup—cakes, cookies, ice cream, candy, ketchup, salad dressing, bread,…the list can go on and on. Likewise with soy. Soybean oil is found everywhere. It is one of the most common cooking oils, especially hydrogenated soybean oil which is used extensively in restaurants and for all types of prepared foods. Like corn, soy in one form or another is found in thousands of consumer products. Canola oil is also widely used in food production and restaurants. With the awareness of the dangers of trans fats from hydrogenated oils, many food producers are turning to canola oil instead. Look at the multitude of the foods that contain sugar. The source of that sugar is most likely GE sugar beets. What about cotton? We don't eat that right? Wrong! Cottonseed oil is a major source of hydrogenated oil used in the food industry. All of these GE crops are also used to feed livestock. The chicken, beef, pork, and even fish we buy at the store are often raised on GE crops. In addition, we are also exposed to GE squash, papaya, and other foods.

Genetic Engineering is an Imprecise Science

Trying to control genetic changes through artificial modification is a dangerous game. It is dangerous because it enables genes to be transferred between species that would never be possible otherwise. Genetic modification involves injecting a gene from one species of plant or animal into a completely different and naturally incompatible species, yielding unexpected and often unpredictable results.

Much of the genetic research that is going on is hidden

from the public because biotech firms require their employees sign legally binding secrecy agreements that forbid them from talking about their research with anyone.

According to geneticist Dr Jonathan Latham, who published an independent study on GE plants, genetic engineering is very imprecise and is making a mess of plant genomes. The process causes unexpected gene mutations and DNA damage. Most GE plants contain more than one genetic modification, some of the plants his team evaluated had as many as 40 different foreign genes in them.[1] Latham says that some of the gene combinations in commercially available plants are so complex that even the biotech companies have given up on trying to assess the potential damage done to the plant's DNA. In other words, even the scientists don't know what they are creating, let alone what effect they will have on our health and the environment.

The insertion of plant, animal, bacterial, and viral genes in food crops can lead to unpredictable and uncontrollable results. Examples of unforeseen changes witnessed in GE foods include poor crop performance, altered nutritional content, increased levels of toxins and allergens in foods, and potential harm to the environment and ecosystems.

Genetically engineered food crops are designed specifically to be resistant to herbicides (such as Monsanto's weed killer Roundup), be resistant to certain pests, or to produce their own insecticide to discourage insect damage. Herbicide resistant crops can withstand exposure to huge doses of chemical weed killers without harm, while indigenous plants nearby wither and die. Plants designed to produce their own toxic chemicals supplement chemical sprays to keep insects at bay. GE crops can contain multiple genetic alternations so that they are resistant to several types of herbicides and produce their own insecticides. Sounds appetizing doesn't it?

As of yet, GE crops are not designed to produce larger plants or be more productive. It's all about managing pests.

Differences in GE and Non-GE Plants

Biotech companies claim that GE crops are no different from conventional crops in nutritional quality and safety. The claim that GE foods are materially comparable to conventional foods, and therefore inherently safe, is false when you consider GE crops are designed to be different.

A recent study published in the journal *Food Chemistry* reveals that there are distinct differences.[2] The researchers analyzed soybeans produced under three separate conditions: (1) genetically modified, glyphosate-tolerant soy, (2) unmodified soy cultivated using a conventional chemical cultivation regime, and (3) unmodified soy produced using an organic cultivation regime.

The researchers stated, "Using 35 different nutritional and elemental variables to characterize each soy sample, we were able to discriminate GM, conventional, and organic soybeans *without exception*, demonstrating *substantial nonequivalence* in compositional characteristics for ready-to-market soybeans." GE soybeans actually had a reduced level of important nutrients and therefore, were less nutritious than conventional soybeans.

Roundup Ready crops are engineered to survive exposure to massive doses that would normally kill the plant as well as all surrounding weeds. As a consequence, GE crops are heavily sprayed, much more so than conventional crops. Even if the nutritional levels were the same, the high level of spraying makes the GE crops less healthful simply because they contain a much higher level of herbicide residue.

Plants that are sprayed with herbicides and insecticides can be taken home and washed or peeled to make them safer because most of the chemical residue clings to the surface of the food.

However, with GE plants, you can't wash out the insecticides that have been placed there genetically because it is in every cell of the plant. It is in what you eat.

Over 37 percent of the GE crops have stacked genes.— two or more GE genes inserted into them. So the plant is not just resistant to Roundup but to other herbicides and may also contain genes to produce their own insecticides. These are the types of GE foods we and the animals in our food supply are being fed.

Environmental Effect

One of the purposes of GE crops is to enable more herbicides to be sprayed on them in order to annihilate all other plants. Roundup is also being used as a desiccant even on conventional crops including wheat and sugar cane, just before harvest. This is because it dries out crops, thus facilitating a more uniform harvest. It also means that we are exposed to a high level of pesticide residue in much of our food.

Herbicides are designed to kill native plants. Tons of herbicides and insecticides are sprayed on farms around the world. Winds, water, rain, and insects spread them throughout the environment, into the soil and water, wreaking havoc wherever they go. It doesn't take a genius to see the tremendous damage these poisons pose to the environment.

With the advent of Roundup Ready crops, use of glyphosate (the active ingredient in Roundup) has significantly risen with about 1 billion pounds sprayed on crops every year. That's 1 billion pounds of herbicide released into the environment annually just from this one product.

Glyphosate's toxicity is well established, with adverse health effects ranging from birth defects to endocrine dysfunction to cancer.[3] Glyphosate is classified as a Class 2A "probable human carcinogen" by the International Agency for Research on Cancer (IARC), a division of the World Health Organization (WHO).

Unbelievably, the US Department of Agriculture (USDA) admits foods are not tested for glyphosate residues due to the high cost of doing such tests. GE crops are heavily contaminated with glyphosate, much more so than conventional crops; this fact alone blows a massive hole in the safety claim.

The increased use of Roundup has caused glyphosate–resistant super weeds to proliferate, leading to a greater use of the herbicides and greater harm to the environment. Current GE crops are being replaced with new varieties that can withstand even heavier doses of herbicides.

Despite the mounting evidence questioning glyphosate's safety, the Environmental Protection Agency (EPA) raised the allowable limits of glyphosate in our food and feed crops. Allowable levels in oilseed crops, such as soy and canola, have been doubled from 20 ppm to 40 ppm. Permissible glyphosate levels in many other foods have been raised by 15 to 25 times previous levels. Root and tuber vegetables got one of the largest boosts, with allowable residue limits being raised form 0.2 ppm to 6.0 ppm. Crops fed to livestock can have much higher levels, up to 400 ppm or more. All GE crops have glyphosate residue. When you eat GE foods, you really can't ignore the fact that you're also eating glyphosate.

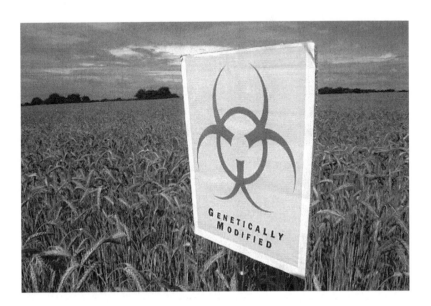

Pesticides and herbicides kill more than just noxious pests, they destroy wildlife that is essential for a healthy environment and food supply. For example, with the increased use of GE crops and massive spraying, Monarch butterfly and honey bee populations have been decimated in the US. It has been estimated that in some areas of the country there has been an 80 percent decline in these important insects within the past few years. This might not sound too alarming, until you consider the impact the absence of just these two insects can have on our lives. Monarch butterflies are pollinators, which makes them important for plant reproduction. They also provide an essential food source for small birds and other animals, which feed larger birds and animals. Monarchs play an important role in ecosystem health and biodiversity. Honey bees too, are pollinators, very important pollinators. Bees are essential for the pollination of numerous flowering plants and food crops. Without them we would lose at least one-third of all our fruits, nuts, and vegetables. It's not just Monarchs and bees that are adversely affected by chemical sprays, but literally millions of insects, animals, and plants as well as humans are harmed by them.

Nearly one billion pounds of Roundup herbicide is used each year for conventional crop production. Genetically engineered crops are more heavily sprayed, since the so-called Roundup Ready crops are designed to survive lethal doses of this chemical, thus increasing the potential harm to the environment. And that is not to mention all of the other herbicides and pesticides that are also used in agriculture.

Soil is the living skin of the earth. Soil is a combination of granulated rock, water, organic matter, and microbes—bacteria, protozoa, fungi, nematodes, and arthropods. One tablespoon of soil contains about 50 billion living organisms. These microorganisms are key in making nutrients available to plants. The nitrogen, potassium, phosphate, calcium, magnesium, and other essential elements are released into the soil by the activity of microorganisms on rocks and organic matter in the soil. Without this great diversity of living creatures in the soil, plants could not exist. Soil organisms are vital to plant health.

Part of what makes fruits and vegetables good for us are the phytonutrients—plant derived nutrients that help protect us from high blood pressure, glaucoma, cancer, premature aging, and other health problems. Phytonutrients are part of the plant's immune system. Organisms in the soil that we might think of as pests actually stimulate plants to make more phytonutrients. So these small stressors actually, in a sense, enhance our health. Being exposed to different organisms improves the health of the plant and improves our health as well.

Pesticides and other agrichemicals not only kill insects but also the beneficial soil microorganisms, degrading soil quality and fertility. This creates a need to use chemical fertilizers, which can cause more harm by further altering the normal soil ecology, making plants more susceptible to disease and pests. This in turn, prompts the use of more agrichemicals and the further reduction of soil productivity, which encourages the use of more chemical fertilizers. The cycle continues, making the soils less and less productive.

Genetic engineering affects livestock as well. GE plants contain their own insecticides to discourage insects and animals from eating them. Farm animals don't like them either and won't touch them if given the choice. Livestock won't eat them unless they are forced to. When GE feed is all that is available, livestock learn to tolerate it or starve. This is just another form of animal cruelty.

When GE crops are planted, there is nothing to prevent the seeds and pollen from being washed or blown to neighboring farms where they can contaminate non-GE crops. What will happen if they crossbreed with native plants? Will the GE gene be passed on? Will heavy spraying cause genetic adaptations in native plants and animals? This has already resulted in the creation of super weeds and super bugs that can withstand pesticide sprays. What will be next?

Will Not Eliminate Hunger

The number one argument and justification for GE crops is the claim that they are needed to prevent starvation and feed the billions of people in the world. Proponents claim GE foods are necessary to feed the world's starving children. Who wouldn't want to do that, right? It's enough to make you want to cry, not because the biotech firms are so benevolent, but because there are people who actually believe this pile of baloney. The one and only reason for GE foods is for profit, pure and simple. There is no intrinsic desire to feed starving people. Their blatant disregard for the health and welfare of people, animals, and the environment is obvious in their refusal to do proper safety and environmental studies and their opposition to independent researchers who desire to undertake such studies. It is also evident in their fierce opposition to labeling of food and their aggressive persecution of farmers who save GE seeds, as they must purchase new seeds annually or face a lawsuit for patent infringement.

The claim that GE crops will eliminate world hunger conveys the idea that they produce a higher yield than conventional crops. However, this is not true. There is no gene in the plants to make them more productive and they are no better than conventional crops at tolerating poor soils or unstable climate conditions. The claim is based solely on the assumption that yields will be better because GE crops are more resistance to herbicides and to bugs eating them.

GE crops have been around for two decades now, if they are going to save the world from starvation, we would already have seen some evidence of that by now, but we haven't. Pesticides that are required on GE crops poison the soil, kill wildlife, and wreak havoc on the ecosystem contributing to the gradual destruction and loss of productive farmland. This would be a disaster if GE crops were grown around the world.

Most people worldwide simply don't want to eat genetically altered foods. As a result, US exports of soy and corn have declined by as much as $300 million per year just from the loss of European exports alone. Corn exports to China dropped 85 percent from 2013 to 1014. How can GE foods feed the world if the world doesn't want to eat them?

Not Proven Safe

Genetic modification of foods has never proven to be safe for humans or the environment. Assessments on safety come only from the biotech corporations themselves, the same companies that profit from these positive safety studies.

Safety studies performed on GE crops fed to animals have generally looked at things such as milk production and meat yield, outcomes that are not relevant to human health. These studies generally do not examine tissues or organs in the animals or look at the biochemistry to identify disease or abnormalities. They are production studies. The vast majority of studies are done to reassure the producers that GE fed animals will live long enough to produce a good yield when they are mature enough to take to market.

There have been very few published studies actually using GE feed. Instead of feeding the test animals GE feed, they just give them the particular proteins the altered plants are suppose to produce. These studies are done using rats. The number of rats used in the studies are too few to produce any real statistically meaningful data. They'll usually observe the rats for only 7 to 14 days, and rarely up to 3 months, and see if the rats die. If they don't, then the GE food containing the protein is declared safe for human consumption regardless of how long or how much a human might consume. We are expected to eat these foods for years, for our entire lives, not just a few days or weeks. However, these proteins, which may come from plants, bacteria, viruses, or animals, can have unknown effects when injected into an entirely different species. There are no long term studies that actually test GE foods. These so-called "safety" studies are used to justify the claim that GE foods are safe for us to eat for an entire lifetime, from birth to death. No additional studies are needed and, therefore, independent researchers need not bother attempting such studies. Consequently, GE seeds are off limits to them. Outside researchers can't even repeat these studies to verify the results.

Another potentially serious consequence of GE foods that has not been investigated is the effect of feeding more than one variety of GE plant. If your diet contains GE corn and soy you could be getting two or more different GE genes. Even a single plant, like corn, can contain more than one foreign gene. The effects of these multiple foreign genes can have a significant effect. In medicine this is referred to polypharmacy—the simultaneous use of two or more drugs.

For example, if you feed somebody an aspirin, the side effects might be so minor it is of little concern. However, if you feed that person another drug at the same time, the two drugs can interact to have very serious consequences. The same can be true with GE foods. We don't know because there have not been any such studies.

Very few real safety studies have been done, primarily because of the difficulty of obtaining GE seeds to study. It is nearly impossible for an independent researcher to get GE seeds to verify the results or to make any meaningful investigation.

Independent researchers who wish to do GE studies are forbidden to use GE crops. It is almost impossible for an independent researcher to obtain GE seeds to do safety studies not authorized or funded (i.e., controlled) by the biotech companies. GE seeds are protected by patent laws. You can't simply go down to your local garden store and purchase the seeds. You must get them directly from the biotech companies. Farmers or anyone else who buys the seeds are required to sign a technology user agreement, which obligates the buyer not do any research on the seeds or give the seeds to anyone else to do research. Such precautions make you wonder why the biotech companies are so afraid of having independent research on their products, are they trying to hide something?

40

Health Dangers of GE Foods

Genetic engineering is not as precise or as accurate as it is generally believed. The genes from foreign organisms are not carefully inserted into the host's DNA at precise locations for optimal function. When scientists inject the gene into the host, they have no control over where the gene may end up on the host's DNA. This is a potentially serious situation as the position the genes occur on the DNA strand can be important. In other words, genetic engineering is like playing Russian Roulette. You don't know what your results will be. The seeds developed from GE may live, and develop much like an ordinary plant, but the chemical changes within the plant are really unknown and could have far reaching effects on our health, especially if they are eaten over a lifetime.

These chemical changes can alter the nutritional content, effect enzyme structure and activity, and produce various compounds that could be toxic. Many plants produce natural toxins to discourage predators (bugs and animals) from eating them. Ordinarily, we can tolerate a small amount of these toxins, an unnatural gene can possibly alter them causing them to be more toxic or more abundant in the plant and thus, harmful for humans and animals. The foreign gene could cause totally new chemicals to be created that could have drastic effects on our health and the health of the environment. Genetic engineering of our foods is really a massive experiment on the human population. We don't know all the dangers. However, some alarming facts have been uncovered.

Despite the difficulties of independent researchers studying GE foods, a very small handful of studies have been done, with alarming results.

One of the first indications that GE foods might be harmful came from the observations of Howard Vlieger, a crop and livestock nutrition advisor.[4] His first experience with genetically modified organisms (GMOs) came in 1997 when he planted a test plot comparing GE corn to the conventional

41

version. He had heard from farmers in Nebraska that cows shied away from the GE corn. So he gave his cows the choice to consume the conventionally grown corn or GE corn. His cows ate the conventionally grown, however they smelled the GE corn and walked away from it. It's not normal for hungry cattle to refuse food. He has tried this with many other animals and found that if they have not been forced to consume GE food in the past, they won't eat it and will go for the conventional feed instead.

In his role as a crop and livestock nutrition adviser, Vlieger knew other farmers who were feeding their animals GE feed. In South Dakota, a farmer fed his sows GE corn and they had on average 1.6 less piglets per litter. The piglets also weighed less at birth.

A farmer from Harlan, Iowa, had sows with pseudo pregnancies. They seemed to be pregnant, but when they delivered, there was only a sack of water, afterbirth, and no pigs. The *Farm Bureau Spokesman* wrote about this farmer's travails and he got calls from other farmers saying they were having the same problem. Interestingly, they were all using the same GE corn. Iowa State University claimed not to find any connection between the GE corn and fertility, but when the farmers stopped using that form of GE corn and switched to conventional corn, the problem disappeared.

Vlieger worked with a hog operation in Nebraska which used GE corn in the feed of breeding animals and found conception rates drop 30 percent. The local vet came out and tested the feed for mycotoxins and mold, but did not find any. The next group of sows was fed conventional corn and conception rates jumped back up to about 90 percent. They switched back to GE corn and conception rates dropped again, this time down by 70 percent.

In Iowa, farmers found anemia and gastrointestinal tract problems such as ileitis (inflammation of the small intestine), bloody bowel, ulcers, and salmonella. When GE corn was taken out of the feed, the problems went away.

42

If GMOs are causing stomach and gastrointestinal inflammation, bloody bowel, ileitis, infertility, ulcers, and false pregnancies in farm animals, *what are they doing to us?* Since glyphosate kills the bacteria in the soil, what does it do to the bacteria inside our bodies and to the environment inside our gastrointestinal tract?

Vlieger's observations sparked Judy Carman, PhD to do an in-depth study with pigs to see if the farmer's experiences were truly related to consuming GE crops. Dr. Carman is an adjunct associate professor at Flinders University in South Australia and the director of the Institute of Health and Environmental Research.[5]

Pigs have a very similar digestive system to humans and what is seen in them when they eat GE foods will likely be found in humans. She wanted to do a proper study with enough pigs to have a statistical significance and for a long enough time to be meaningful. Her first obstacle to overcome was legally obtaining GE seeds. The biotech companies would not sell them to her for her study so she had to devise a means to get them another way. After a great deal of effort, she was able to acquire seeds legally for her study. She declines to reveal how she obtained the seeds because she does not want that loophole to be plugged.

She and her colleagues obtained piglets as soon as they were weaned. The first solid food they were given was either GE or non-GE. The pigs were fed for their entire commercial lifespan. This was a commercial piggery study, it was done under commercial piggery conditions. The animals, once they reached 5 months were processed according to industry standards. So the pigs were exposed to the GE feed for less than 5 months.

Unlike industry sponsored studies that use only a handful of rats, she used a total of 168 pigs in her study, enough to derive some statistical significance in the results.

Carman's study found many of the same problems reported by Vlieger. There was a significant increase in stomach inflammation in the pigs—severe inflammation. "When I say 'severe,' I'm talking about a stomach that is swollen and cherry red in color over almost the entire surface of the stomach," says Carman. "This is not the sort of stomach that you or I would want to have at all."

They next looked at reproductive health. They couldn't examine male reproductive health because all the boars were neutered at 3 days of age. But they could examine the female pigs. They found an abnormal thickening of the uterus in the pigs fed GE food. The uterus was 25 percent heavier. In the paper they talk about all of the disease states that this could represent.[6]

Your body houses some 100 trillion bacteria. You have more bacteria in your body than you have cells, 10 times more. In essence, we are a colony of microbes. These organisms are not simply freeloaders feeding off our bodies, but work in harmony with our bodies performing a wide variety of important functions essential for good health. The type of bacteria in your gastrointestinal (GI) tract is just as important as your own cells for proper digestive function. Some bacteria produce essential vitamins for us, other help us digest foods or strengthen our immune system. Some microbes, including viruses and yeasts, can be harmful and wreak havoc on our bodies if their numbers get out of hand. Having large populations of so-called "friendly" bacteria prevent the overgrowth of potentially harmful microbes. Without these tiny organisms we could not exist, with the wrong type we become prone to malnutrition and disease. Having the right proportions of the different bacteria and other microbes helps keep us healthy.

One of the very serious dangers of GE crops is the alteration of the gut microbiota—the microorganisms living in your GI tract. The studies by Howard Vlieger and Judy Carman demonstrated that diets containing GM foods lead to severe GI inflammation and damage. While it is possible that something in the GM foods could be irritating the GI tract causing these conditions, another possibility is that the high percentage of glyphosate residue on these foods is causing it. We know glyphosate kills soil bacteria, why not gut bacteria as well? These GE chemicals and herbicides could be killing the beneficial gut bacteria, allowing more virulent strains to proliferate, creating an environment in the gut leading to inflammation, leaky gut, ulcers, bleeding, immune disorders, allergies, nutrient malabsorption, and reduced nutrient syntheses, among other things.

Another rare study by an independent researcher was conducted by Dr. Gilles-Eric Seralini. He replicated the studies that the industry used to establish the safety of the GE foods. But rather than terminating the study at three months or less, he took it to two years, which is the typical life expectancy of a rat. In order to obtain statistical significance, Seralini's study included 200 rats, unlike the typical 10 or 20 used in biotech supported studies.

There were some very significant differences between Seralini's study and the previous industry-sponsored studies. Rats fed GE food their entire lives developed huge breast tumors and suffered from liver and kidney damage. As much

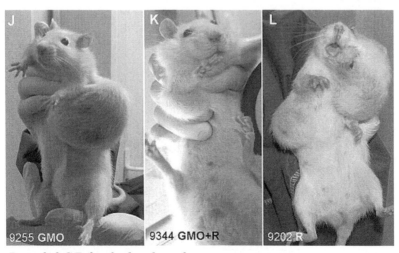

Rats fed GE foods developed enormous tumors.

as 80 percent of the female rats developed large tumors by the beginning of the 24th month, with up to three tumors per animal. Up to 70 percent of female rats died prematurely. Large tumors began to appear after only seven months. However, the majority of tumors were detectable only after 18 months, meaning they could be discovered only in long-term feeding trials.

Since Roundup sprayed foods are always contaminated with residual glyphosate the effect may possibly have been due to the herbicide rather than the genetic alternation. To identify this possibility Seralini separated the rats into groups. He fed one group of rats GE food and a second group non-GE food, both without glyphosate contamination.. Another two groups were fed either GE or non-GE foods that were sprayed with glyphosate. He found that there were problems with animals fed the glyphosate and with those fed the non-sprayed GE food, but when glyphosate was combined with GE crops, the effects were worse.[7]

Digestive disorders are becoming rampant—sensitivity to wheat and gluten, celiac disease, food allergies, Crohn's, colitis, and GERD. Such conditions appear to be epidemic. Food allergies are becoming more common. Reproductive health is becoming a growing concern. Infertility, miscarriages, premature births, cesarean deliveries, birth defects, and childhood developmental disorders are at an all time high. Cancer is the second leading cause of death. We've been at war with cancer for over 40 years and are losing the battle. Are GE crops and pesticides to blame? Until the biotech companies allow independent researchers to do meaningful safety studies we won't know for sure, but the evidence so far suggests it may be so.

In the meantime, we can support efforts to label GE foods so that we know what we are buying at the store. At this point, the only guarantee that your food is safe is to buy and eat organically raised foods or grow your own.

Chapter 5

Monsanto's Roundup: It's Enough to Make You Sick

Monsanto, the maker of Roundup herbicide, is hiding the truth about the dangers of glyphosate, the active ingredient in Roundup, and trying to paint a picture of it being essential for agriculture and feeding the world without any harmful impact on the environment or our health. It is so safe, they claim, that it can be used in residential areas. Nothing could be further from the truth. Monsanto, has falsified data on Roundup's safety, and marketed it to park departments and consumers claiming it to be "environmentally friendly," "biodegradable," and that it "leaves the soil clean," to encourage its use on roadsides, playgrounds, golf courses, schoolyards, lawns, and home gardens. This claim was recently challenged in a French court and Monsanto was found guilty of false advertising.

Dr. Stephanie Seneff, a research scientist at the Massachusetts Institute of Technology (MIT), says glyphosate is possibly "the most important factor in the development of multiple chronic diseases and conditions that have become prevalent in Westernized societies." Including, but not limited to, infertility, gastrointestinal diseases (Crohn's, colitis, IBS), allergies, cancer, cardiovascular disease, multiple sclerosis, Alzheimer's, Parkinson's, and autism.[1]

One of the ways glyphosate harms our bodies is by killing the good bacteria that inhabit our gastrointestinal tract. These bacteria are essential for proper digestive and immune function as well as our overall health. Monsanto has emphatically claimed that Roundup is harmless to animals and humans because the way it kills weeds is by interfering with the shikimate pathway—a metabolic process whereby plants produce amino acids which are essential for plant growth and development. This process is absent in all animals. That may sound convincing, but the shikimate pathway is also used by bacteria, fungi, and algae. Therefore, glyphosate is deadly to soil organisms, degrading the productivity of our farmland, and to our gut bacteria which are essential to our health and to the health of all animals. In this way, Roundup is destroying the health of all humans and animals exposed to this herbicide. Glyphosate also disrupts enzymatic activity in animals and humans. Certain enzymes that play a crucial role in neutralizing toxins are deactivated by glyphosate. This means that environmental chemicals and poisons, including Roundup, become even more toxic.[2]

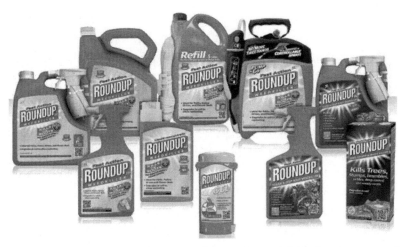

Roundup is the most commonly used pesticide for home and commercial use.

Researchers have found that Roundup itself is even more toxic than glyphosate alone. The reason for this is that Roundup includes other chemicals besides glyphosate. One of these is a surfactant, TN-20, which greatly enhances the toxic effects of glyphosate. Animal studies have shown that the combination of TN-20 and glyphosate leads to cell damage, degeneration, and death at concentrations where neither substance working alone would show this effect.[3]

In humans, prolonged skin exposure to glyphosate-surfactant herbicide has been shown to produce local swelling, blistering, and exuding wounds, followed by neurological impairment and reduced nerve function. It is apparent that Roundup is not as safe as Monsanto claims it to be.

It's Not Just in the Food

Since genetically engineered (GE) crops are heavily sprayed with Roundup, they are also heavily contaminated with it as well. Every time we eat foods containing GE products we are ingesting glyphosate. What's even worse is that this poison is released into the environment where people and animals can be exposed to much larger doses. The consequences can be staggering.

In Argentina the introduction of GE crops and pesticide spraying is turning into a nightmare. Argentine laborer Fabian Tomasi was never trained to handle pesticides. His job was to keep the crop-dusters flying by filling their tanks as quickly as possible. "I prepared millions of liters of poison without any kind of protection, no gloves, masks, or special clothing," he said. "I didn't know anything." For three years, Tomasi was routinely exposed to chemicals as he pumped pesticides into the tanks of crop-dusters. Now, at the age of 47 he's a living skeleton and near death from polyneuropathy, a debilitating neurological disorder, which has left him wasted and shriveled.

Schoolteacher Andrea Druetta lives in Santa Fe Province, the heart of Argentina's soy country, where agrochemical

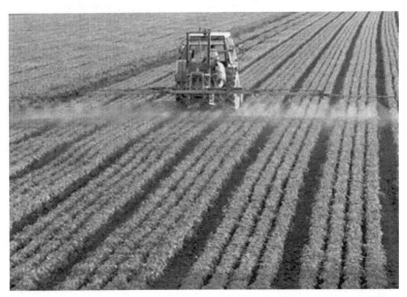

Fields of soybeans being sprayed. According to the USDA, more than 90 percent of the soybeans grown on US farms are genetically engineered to tolerate herbicides, nearly all of them Roundup.

spraying is banned within 500 meters (550 yards) of populated areas. But soy is planted just 30 meters (33 yards) from her back door. Homes, as well as schools in the area, are often exposed to Roundup spray from planes that come too close and from winds that blow the pesticide their way. Druetta filed complaints with the city, alleging that several students fainted when pesticides drifted into their classrooms and that their tap water is contaminated. She said, a neighbor keeps a freezer of rabbit and bird carcasses, hoping someone will test them to see why they dropped dead after the spraying.

After Sofia Gatica lost her newborn to kidney failure, she filed a complaint that led to Argentina's first criminal convictions for not following safety regulations while spraying. But the verdict came too late for many of her 5,300 neighbors. A government study there found alarming levels of agrochemical contamination in the soil and drinking water, and 80 percent of the children surveyed carried traces of glyphosate in their blood.

Argentina is the world's third-largest soybean producer, however, the chemicals powering this boom aren't confined to just soy but are sprayed on cotton, corn, and other GE crops. A nation once known for its grass-fed beef has undergone a remarkable transformation since 1996, when Monsanto promised that adopting its GE seeds and chemicals would increase crop yields and lower pesticide use. Today, Argentina's entire soy crop and nearly all its corn and cotton are genetically modified, with soy cultivation alone tripling to 47 million acres (19 million hectares).

Despite Monsanto's claim (i.e, lie) that GE seeds would reduce pesticide use, it has dramatically increased it (to the benefit of Monsanto, which sells both the GE seed and the pesticides). Pesticide use in the country increased from just 9 million gallons in 1990 to more than 84 million gallons by 2013.

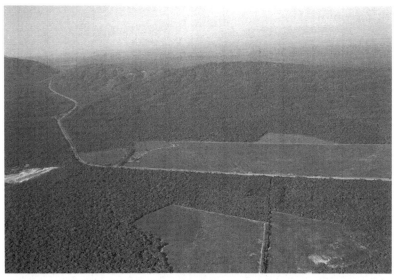

Argentina's forests are disappearing to make room for soybean cultivation. Today only 30 percent of the country's original forests remain.

Overall, Argentine farmers apply an estimated 4.3 pounds of pesticides per acre, more than twice what US farmers use. The spray drifts into schools and homes and settles over water sources; farm workers mix poisons with no protective gear; villagers store water in pesticide containers that should have been destroyed.

This isn't just a problem in Argentina, it's happening in other countries too, especially throughout South America. Argentina, Brazil, Paraguay, Uruguay, and Bolivia are among the top 10 ten soybean producers in the world. Brazil alone produces nearly 16 times more soy than Canada, another country in the top 10.

Growing Health Problem

Now doctors are warning that uncontrolled pesticide applications could be the cause of growing health problems among the 12 million people who live in Argentina's vast farm belt.

In Santa Fe, cancer rates are two to four times higher than the national average. In Chaco, birth defects have quadrupled in the past decade since spraying become more prevalent.

"The change in how agriculture is produced has brought, frankly, a change in the profile of diseases," says Dr. Medardo Avila Vazquez, a pediatrician and neonatologist. "We've gone from a pretty healthy population to one with a high rate of cancer, birth defects, and illnesses seldom seen before."

Molecular biologist Dr. Andres Carrasco at the University of Buenos Aires says the use of glyphosate pesticides (Roundup) is worrisome and could spell trouble for human health. He found that injecting a very low dose of glyphosate into embryos can change levels of retinoic acid, causing the same sort of spinal defects in frogs and chickens that doctors increasingly are registering in communities where farm chemicals are used.

Retinoic acid, a form of vitamin A, is fundamental for keeping cancers in check and triggering genetic expression, the process by which embryonic cells develop into organs and limbs.

"If it's possible to reproduce this in a laboratory, surely what is happening in the field is much worse," Carrasco said. His findings, published in the journal *Chemical Research* in Toxicology in 2010[4], were rebutted by Monsanto. "Glyphosate is even less toxic than the [insect] repellent you put on your children's skin," said Pablo Vaquero, Monsanto's corporate affairs director in Buenos Aires. Tell that to Fabian Tomasi who lays in a bed at home dying from exposure to the pesticide; or to Andrea Druetta whose students fainted when exposed to wind-blown spray; or Sofia Gatica whose infant died of kidney failure after exposure; and to all the dead rabbits and birds littering the fields after spraying.

In response to soaring complaints, Argentina's President, Cristina Fernandez, ordered a commission in 2009 to study the impact of agrochemical spraying on human health. Its initial report called for "systematic controls over concentrations of herbicides and their compounds...such as exhaustive laboratory and field studies involving formulations containing glyphosate as well as its interactions with other agrochemicals as they are actually used in our country." But the commission hasn't met since 2010, the auditor general found. Some have speculated that the members of the commission have been bribed to sit back and do nothing. In the meantime, Monsanto earns millions of dollars in seed and pesticide sales.

Dr. Damian Verzenassi, who directs the Environment and Health program at the National University of Rosario's medical school, decided to try to figure out what was behind an increase in cancer, birth defects and miscarriages in Argentina's hospitals.

"We didn't set out to find problems with agrochemicals. We went to see what was happening with the people," he said.

Since 2010, this house-to-house epidemiological study has reached 65,000 people in Santa Fe province, finding cancer rates two to four times higher than the national average, including breast, prostate and lung cancers. Researchers also found high rates of thyroid disorders and chronic respiratory illness.

Dr. Maria del Carmen Seveso, who has spent 33 years running intensive care wards and ethics committees in Chaco province, became alarmed at regional birth reports showing a quadrupling of congenital defects, from 19.1 per 10,000 to 85.3 per 10,000 in the decade after genetically modified crops and their agrochemicals were approved in Argentina.

Determined to find out why, she and her colleagues surveyed 2,051 people in six towns in Chaco, and found significantly more diseases and defects in villages surrounded by industrial agriculture than in those surrounded by cattle ranches. In Avia Terai, 31 percent said a family member had cancer in the past 10 years, compared with 3 percent in the ranching village of Charadai.

The survey found diseases Seveso said were uncommon before—birth defects including malformed brains, exposed spinal cords, blindness and deafness, neurological damage, infertility, and strange skin problems.

Aixa Cano, a shy 5-year-old, has hairy moles all over her body. Her neighbor, 2-year-old Camila Veron, was born with multiple organ problems and is severely disabled. Doctors told their mothers that agrochemicals may be to blame.

"They told me that the water made this happen because they spray a lot of poison here," said Camila's mother, Silvia Achaval. "People who say spraying poison has no effect, I don't know what sense that has because here you have the proof," she added, pointing at her daughter.

It's nearly impossible to prove that exposure to a specific chemical caused an individual's cancer or birth defect. But like the other doctors, Seveso said their findings should prompt a rigorous government investigation. Instead, their 68-page report was shelved for a year by Chaco's health ministry.

Again, government corruption and bribes stalled any progress toward resolving this growing health problem. A year later, a leaked copy was posted on the Internet.

How Tropical Oils Can Protect Us

The most common GE crops in the US, Canada, and elsewhere are soybeans, corn, canola, and cottonseed—all of which are used to make editable oils. The cooking oils, shortenings, and margarines you purchase at the grocery store, the oils used in most all of the packaged, canned, and frozen foods you buy, and the oils used in the vast majority of restaurants come from GE crops. The oils in our diet are the most prevalent source of GE foods in our diet.

In the US and many other countries there currently are no laws that require food manufacturers to identify on the labels of their products that they contain GE ingredients. How do you avoid these oils? One way is to purchase "certified organic" products. Organically raised crops, by definition, are those that have been raised and processed without exposure to pesticides and other chemicals. Since GE crops are designed specifically to survive heavy doses of pesticides, they are naturally heavily sprayed. Therefore, no GE ingredients should be in a certified organic product. Be aware that the word "Natural" on a label does not mean organic. This term has no official meaning, so any product can use the word "Natural" regardless of where the ingredients come from or how they are produced.

If you are mindful of the types of fats and oils you use, you can avoid all of the oils that are tainted with GE ingredients, even if the product is not certified organic. Oils that are safe to use include extra virgin olive oil, avocado oil, macadamia nut oil, coconut oil, palm oil (including red palm oil), and palm kernel oil. These oils are not derived from GE sources and are completely safe to use. Many of them, like coconut oil and palm oil, are generally organically grown, and therefore, free from pesticide residue, even if they are not labeled "organic," since they are often produced by farmers who do not use any pesticides or chemicals.

It is sad that the people of Argentina and other countries that grow GE crops are suffering from the effects of the chemicals used in modern biotech farming. Instead of growing soy, corn, canola, or cottonseed, they could be growing coconut or palm, which are not genetically engineered, vastly more environmentally safe, and far healthier. All commercially available brands and types of coconut and palm oil are GE free.

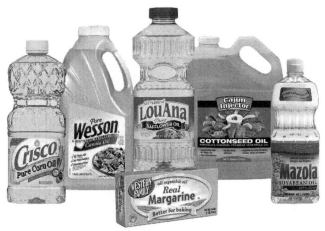

Oils that are commonly produced using genetically modified plants.

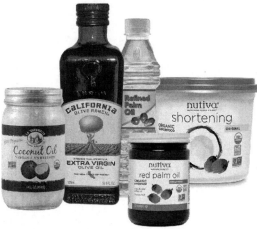

Oils that are never produced from genetically modified plants.

Chapter 6

The Soy Deception: How Seed Oils are Destroying the Rainforests

The Attack on the Tropical Oils

During the 1970s and 1980s the soybean industry was troubled by emerging evidence that soybean oil consumption lowered immunity, increased susceptibility to infectious disease, and promoted cancer.

At this same time saturated fats were being scrutinized because of their tendency, in general, to raise blood cholesterol levels. The bigwigs in the soybean industry got the bright idea that if they could demonize the competition, by making saturated fats appear to be the cause of heart disease—the nation's number one killer—people wouldn't pay much attention to the negative findings coming out about soybean oil. Starting in the mid-1980s the soybean industry began a multi-million dollar anti-saturated fat campaign. Saturated fats increased cholesterol, they said, and high cholesterol causes heart disease. The tropical oils (coconut, palm, and palm kernel oils) were singled out as being the worst offenders because of their high saturated fat content.

Some, but not all, saturated fats do raise total cholesterol, but there was no solid evidence that high cholesterol actually caused heart disease. That is why high cholesterol is only considered a "risk factor" rather than a cause. But that didn't stop the soy industry. Gullible consumer advocate groups like The Center for Science in the Public Interest (CSPI) and The American Heart Savers Association were swayed by the misleading information and began their own campaigns against saturated fats.[1] In these groups the soybean industry found very vocal, high profile allies which spearheaded much of the criticism against saturated fats, and particularly against the tropical oils. These organizations placed anti-saturated fat ads in the media, published newsletters and magazine articles, and books, and lobbied for political action against the use of tropical oils and other saturated fats.

The soybean industry fed misleading information to these groups and allowed them to fight the battle. The soybean industry took a back seat and stayed out of the limelight. This was very clever from a marketing perspective because now the soybean industry wasn't viewed as openly attacking their competition. Since the bulk of the attack came from supposedly impartial third parties, their message had more impact. People were swayed against saturated fats and the tropical oils.

Restaurants and food manufacturers sensitive to customer fear of saturated fats, began removing these fats from their foods and replacing them with vegetable oils. Tropical oil consumption plummeted while soybean oil sales skyrocketed. In the United States soybean oil soon accounted for about 80 percent of all the vegetable oil consumed.

During this time, one thing the soybean industry conveniently neglected to tell the public was that the saturated fats were not being replaced with ordinary vegetable oil, but by *hydrogenated* soybean oil! Hydrogenated soybean oil contains toxic trans fatty acids and is far more damaging to the heart than *any* other fat. It has also been linked to numerous other health problems including diabetes, cancer, and various autoimmune diseases. In terms of health, it is absolutely the worse fat that could be used.

58

The soy industry was aware of many of the detrimental effects associated with hydrogenated vegetable oils and trans fatty acids, that is why it was never publicly announced that saturated fat would eventually be replaced by hydrogenated vegetable oils. They succeeded in demonizing all saturated fats, including healthy coconut and palm oils, for the sake of profit. The plan was an overwhelming financial success. Over the next two decades hydrogenated vegetable oils found their way into over 50 percent of all the foods on supermarket shelves, amounting to about 40,000 different products. Hydrogenated soybean oil consumption dramatically increased, so did numerous diseases now found to be associated trans fatty acids.

In recent years, however, coconut and palm oils have been making a comeback. Careful review of previous research and more current medical studies have exonerated the tropical oils from the claim that they promote heart disease. In fact, if anything, they appear to help protect against heart disease as well as many of the other diseases now known to be linked to hydrogenated vegetable oils.

With the growing awareness of the dangers of trans fatty acids in hydrogenated vegetable oils and the landmark announcement in 2002 from the United States Institute of Medicine stating that "no level of trans fatty acids is safe in the diet," tropical oils are returning. Coconut and palm oils are naturally trans fat free. Palm oil in particular has enjoyed a resurgence internationally as a preferred cooking oil. Its excellent stability and high smoke point make it ideal for cooking and frying. In terms of health, it is far superior to hydrogenated soybean oil.

Many restaurants and food manufacturers are now replacing their hydrogenated soybean and cottonseed oils with palm oil. Consequently, hydrogenated vegetable oil sales are declining. The soybean and seed oil industries are alarmed. In an effort to protect their profits they've returned to their old tried and true means of demonizing the competition in order to make their products more acceptable.

The War on Palm Oil

Relying on old friends, such as CSPI, a new wave of attacks have been focused on palm oil. CSPI reverting back to its old standard of trying to create fear in the minds of the public, continues to harp on the saturated fat issue. They have even published full page ads in the *New York Times* suggesting that palm oil is worse than hydrogenated soybean oil. The impact the CSPI has had with this approach has generally been flat. Too many people now are aware of the benefits of the tropical oils and the dangers of hydrogenated vegetable oils. Their anti-saturated fat rhetoric isn't having the same impact as it did in previous years. There is just too much scientific evidence to refute their unfounded claims.

Desperate to find an alternative means of attack, the seed oil industry has found a new ally in green groups such as Friends of the Earth, Greenpeace, and WWF, highly vocal politically active environmental groups. Fueled by support and misleading data from the soy and seed oil industries, the green groups have now waged a war against palm oil on the grounds that palm cultivation is destroying the environment. They claim that rainforests are being leveled to make room for palm plantations, destroying the ecology and bringing endangered species, such as the orangutan, to the brink of extinction. Anyone with any sense of responsibility for the environment would be emotionally swayed by this argument.

The problem, however, is that it's not true. Like a magician, the soybean industry is a master of illusion. They were successful in creating the illusion that tropical oils caused heart disease and that hydrogenated soybean oils were a better option. Now that we have discovered the secret to that illusion, they are trying to trick us again. This time they are attempting to create an illusion that their competition is harming the environment while they, on the other hand, are environmentally friendly. In reality, the soybean and seed oil industries are causing more destruction to the environment than probably any other agricultural industry on the planet.

In North America the attack against palm oil is headed by the soybean industry and their friends. In Europe it is fueled by the seed oil industry. The European Commission (EC) is funding millions to green groups each year so that green groups are campaigning against palm oil (in the guise to save orangutans). But the real agenda behind the curtain is that the European Commission wants to sabotage the palm oil industry so that Europe can sell their rapeseed, linseed, canola, and sunflower oils.

Green groups have been spreading the seed oil industries' lies about palm oil for years. They claim that the orangutans are being killed deliberately in Malaysia and Indonesia for palm oil. Not so. It is already illegal under Malaysian law to kill orangutans, with hefty penalties for those that violate the law. Therefore, the push for a "no-kill" policy is absurd.

Recently, the Italian organization Libertiamo, exposed the real truth about the anti-palm oil campaigns in Europe.

Fact 1: The European Commission has been sponsoring millions of dollars each year to green groups to campaign aggressively against palm oil. The EC has paid nearly 5 million Euros to the World Wildlife Fund (WWF), 4 million Euros to Friends of the Earth, and 1 million Euros to Climate Action Network (Can).[2] The EC is determined to protect at all cost, their own indigenous edible oil industry that cannot compete with palm oil!

Fact 2: Green group's anti-palm oil campaigns are not based on facts but aimed at spreading exaggerated lies about orangutans and deforestation. Green groups falsely claim that rainforest deforestation in Borneo is happening at 300 football fields per hour! Really? 7,200 football fields a day? They also claim that up to 5,000 orangutans are killed each year to make room for oil palm. Over the past 10 years that would amount to 50,000 orangutans being killed. Are there really that many orangutans in Borneo? If such were the case, would they really be considered endangered? Exaggeration and fabrication. When confronted to debate the facts, these green groups say, "We are not a research organization." In other words, don't cloud the issue with facts, we don't want to hear it.

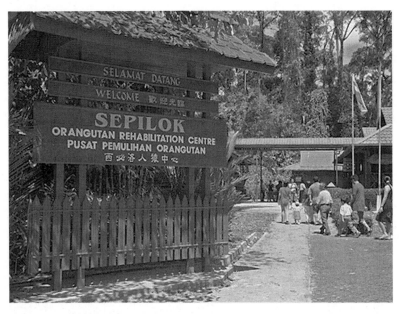

This is Sepilok Orangutan Rehabilitation Centre in Sabah Malaysia. It has a huge rainforest reserve and protects the orangutans. Orangutans are fed every day and cared for by rangers in the protected rainforest. Will the green groups show you these campaigns? No. Because, according to Liberatiamo, they are paid by the EC to brainwash the public to be anti-palm oil.

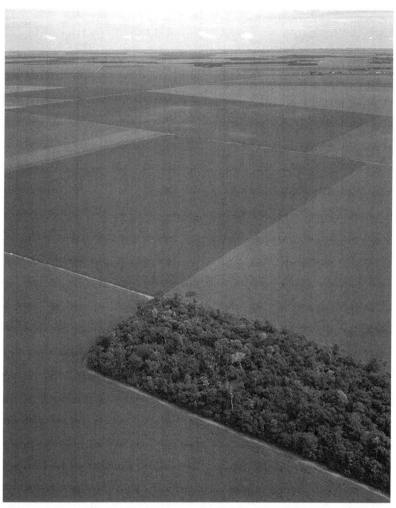

Thousands upon thousands of acres of rainforest are cleared each year for soybean cultivation. Note, there are no oil palms growing here, the deforested area is covered in soy.

Fact 3: Activists and green groups are calling to boycott products that contain palm oil in an attempt to harm companies that use palm oil and force them to stop. Such a concentrated effort against a single ingredient has never been seen before. The organized effort against a truly harmful product like hydrogenated oils was never so aggressive.

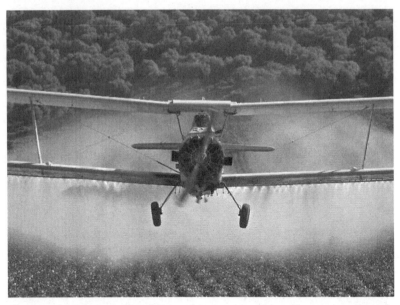

Soybeans, especially GE soybeans, are heavily sprayed with pesticides. Note the spray blowing into the forest in the background. Soybean cultivation not only strips rainforests bare, but poisons all of the surrounding vegetation and wildlife, doing far more harm to the environment than oil palms could. You can bet the owners of this field aggressively kill any animals that may wander into the fields or pose any threat to the soybean crop.

Fact 4: The anti-palm oil campaign is the most aggressive in Europe, America, and Australia–all countries that are planting soybeans, corn, and canola, vying to wrestle for market share from palm oil.

The media is quick to latch onto shocking and emotion-gripping stories about the harm caused by oil palm operations. For instance, a British newspaper reported along with a photo that a baby orangutan was kept in a small cage all his life. Shocking? Yes. True? No! The story was false.

Malaysian news reported that the baby orangutan was actually being transported from a medical center back to the forest after receiving medical treatment!

Once the story was exposed as a fraud, did the British press publish an apology? None whatsoever! The story continued to be spread on the Internet and elsewhere as if it were true.

Loving orangutans is ethical. But using it as a disguise for the agenda of trade war, spreading lies to destroy the palm oil industry for profit of soybean, canola, and sunflower oil industries, while making Asia's farming population poorer, now that is very unethical.

The Amazon Crisis

In the time it takes to read this book, hundreds of acres of Brazil's Amazon rainforest will have been destroyed, much of it for soybean cultivation. Thousands of acres of land around the world are being plowed under to raise soybeans, corn, canola, cottonseed, and sunflower for oil production.

Brazil holds about 30 percent of the Earth's remaining tropical rainforest. The Amazon Basin produces roughly 20 percent of the Earth's oxygen, creates much of its own rainfall, and harbors many unknown species. The Brazilian rainforest is the world's most biologically diverse habitat. Close to 20 percent of the Amazon rainforest has already been cut down.

Now, industrial-scale soybean producers are joining loggers and cattle ranchers, speeding up destruction and further fragmenting the great Brazilian wilderness. Between the years 2000 and 2005, Brazil lost more than 50,000 square miles of rainforest. A large portion of that was for soybean farming.[3]

Soybean production in the Brazilian Amazon soared after heat-tolerant varieties were introduced in 1997. In just ten years, exports of soybeans grown in the Amazon Basin have reached 42 million tons a year. Total annual soybean production in Brazil is about 85 million tons. Brazil will soon surpass the United States as the world's leader in soybean production.

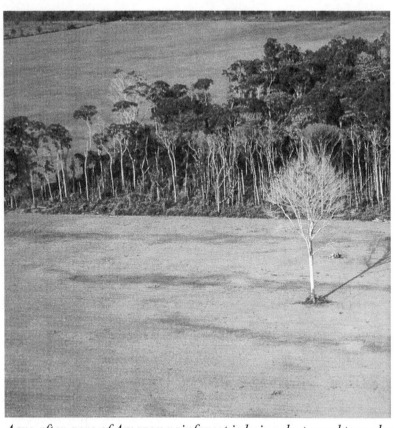

Acre after acre of Amazon rainforest is being destroyed to make room for soybean cultivation, leaving the land scarred, the soil and water polluted, and forcing indigenous peoples off their land.

At the current rate of clearing, scientists predict that 40 percent of the Amazon will be destroyed and a further 20 percent degraded within two decades. If that happens, the forest's ecology will begin to unravel. Intact, the Amazon produces half its own rainfall through the moisture it releases into the atmosphere. Eliminate enough of that rain through clearing, and the remaining trees dry out and die. Currently trees are being wantonly burned to create open land for soybean cultivation. Consequently, Brazil has become one of the world's largest emitters of greenhouse gases.

There are few paved roads into the Amazon. The most controversial is the 1,100 mile long BR-163 highway which runs straight into the heart of the Amazon Basin providing an alleyway for industrial-sized soybean operations to grab up millions of acres of land. Because of the thousands of tons of soy transported over this road it is nicknamed the "soy highway."

The decimation of the Amazon is, for the most part, done legally. Even the governor of the state of Mato Gross, on the edge of the Amazon Basin is a part of it. Governor Blairo Maggi is the world's largest single soybean producer, growing 350,000 acres. That's equivalent to 547 square miles of Amazon rainforest that has been leveled for soybean production. His is just one of many industrial-sized soybean operations in the area. In 2005 Greenpeace awarded Maggi the Golden Chain Saw award for his role in leveling the rainforest.

Clearing the land for soybean production is only part of the problem. Soybean cultivation destroys habitat for wildlife including endangered or unknown species. It increases greenhouse gases, which are believed to contribute to global warming and disrupts the life of indigenous tribes who depend on the forest for food and shelter. Soybeans need large amounts of acid-neutralizing lime, as well as fertilizers, pesticides, and herbicides. All of which are creating an environmental hazard. Toxic chemicals contaminate the forest, poison rivers, and destroy wildlife. Indigenous native communities complain about poisoned water and dying fish.

The environmental destruction caused by soybean farming isn't limited to the Amazon, it occurs throughout the world wherever soybeans are produced. That's hundreds of thousands of acres of deforestation, over cultivation and destruction of the land, and billions of tons of toxic chemicals spewed into the environment year after year, contaminating our soils, water, and destroying wildlife, not to mention what it is doing to us. Genetically modified soy was specifically developed to withstand the toxins so farmers could spray even more pesticides on them without diminishing yields. Talk about destroying the environment, the soybean industry has to rank near the top of the offender's list.

How Palm Oil is Feeding the World and Protecting the Planet

Now, let's take a look at the palm oil industry. When you compare soy cultivation to that of palm, there is a huge difference. Palm cultivation is perhaps, the world's most environmentally friendly commercial crop. After oil palms reach maturity they are commercially productive for at least a quarter of a century. That means that once the trees are planted, the soil remains essentially undisturbed for decades. Unlike soy, were the ground is dug up and recultivated every year, year after year. Among oil palms native grasses and scrubs are allowed to repopulate the space between trees. The natural habitat returns, complete with wildlife. An oil palm plantation takes on the appearance of a rainforest, filled with vegetation. Wild boar, monkeys, birds, and other wildlife are allowed to roam in and out of the plantations, just as they do in the wild. Chemical fertilizers and pesticides are rarely, if ever, used. Since the ground is continually covered with trees and growth, the soil is not eroded, maintaining the integrity of the environment from the tiniest soil organisms to the largest land animals. So a palm plantation blends into the environment without causing untold disruption.

Compare that with a soybean plantation where all trees and other vegetation are killed and removed. Only soybeans are allowed to grow. And what about wildlife? Animals would trample or eat the crops, so they are fenced out, shot, or poisoned.

Unlike soy and most other crops that produce once a year, oil palms produce fruit year round, so they are always in season. This allows for a high yield of fruit on comparatively

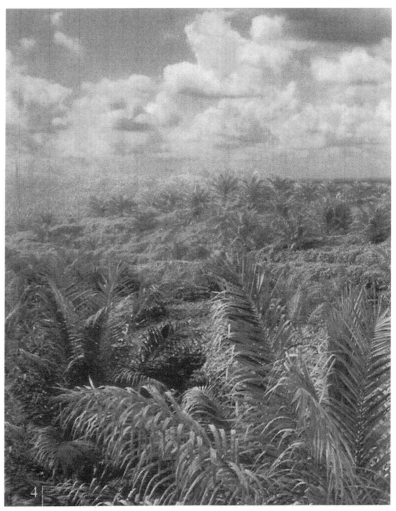

Palm plantations are like thick forests filled with plant growth and wildlife. Much greener than soybean or canola farms, don't you agree?

little acreage. For this reason, *the oil palm produces more oil per acre than any other vegetable source.* For example, in one year on one acre of land a farmer can produce 18 gallons of corn oil, or 35 gallons of cottonseed oil, or 48 gallons of soybean oil. However, on the same amount of land you can

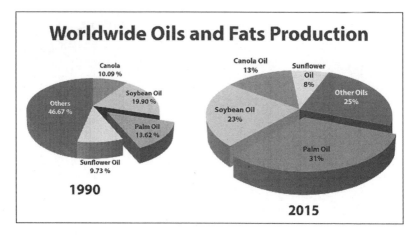

Worldwide Oils and Fats Production

1990
- Canola 10.09 %
- Others 46.67 %
- Soybean Oil 19.90 %
- Palm Oil 13.62 %
- Sunflower Oil 9.73 %

2015
- Canola Oil 13%
- Sunflower Oil 8%
- Other Oils 25%
- Soybean Oil 23%
- Palm Oil 31%

produce *635 gallons* of palm oil! No, that is not a misprint. You read that correctly, 635 gallons of palm oil compared to just 48 gallons of soybean oil. In terms of land use, you would need to plant 13 acres of soy or 35 acres of corn to produce an equal amount of oil from just one acre of palm.

So, soybean cultivation requires 13 times more land to produce the same amount of oil. And this land is stripped of all other vegetation, and continually plowed and replowed, and poisoned with pesticides. While oil palms are planted once and then the land is allowed to return mostly to its natural state without harming the environment.

Until just a few years ago, more soybean oil was produced annually worldwide than any other oil. It has now dropped to second place behind palm oil. What that means is that millions of acres of land has and still is being destroyed for soybean cultivation. More land, like that in the Amazon Basin, is being leveled and forests and wildlife habitat being destroyed to meet the high demand for soybean oil. Replacing soybean oil with palm oil, is not only a healthier option, but would save countless acres of land from untold environmental damage. In the Amazon we have no idea how many rare species of plants and animals are becoming extinct in the name of corporate profit.

Oil Palm vs Other Major Oil Crops

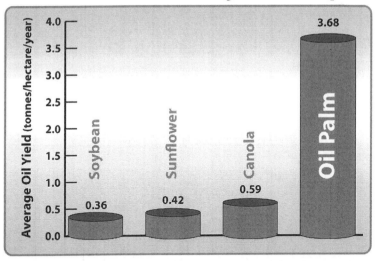

Oil palm is the world's most efficient oil-bearing crop in terms of land utilization, efficiency, and productivity. A single hectare of land produces about 10 times more oil than other oilseeds. Globally oil palm produces just as much oil as soy, yet utilizes only one-tenth the land area.

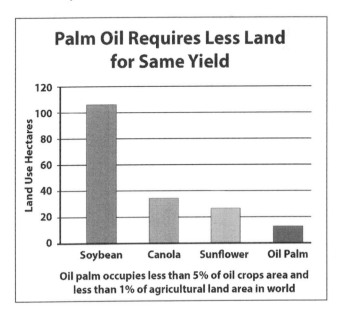

Performance of Oil Palm vs Soybean in CO2 Sequestration

Oil Crop	Oil Palm	Soybean
Total Global Planted Area (mil ha)	9.16	92.54
O2 Released (mil tonne)	195.1	236.9
Co2 Absorbed (mil tonne)	268.4	325.7
Average O2 Released (t/ha)	21.3	2.56
Average Co2 Absorbed (t/ha)	29.3	3.52

Oil palm helps protect against global warming. Total area globally devoted to oil palm production is 9.16 million hectares (35,367 sq miles). Total land area under soybean cultivation is 92.54 million hectares (357, 299 sq miles), more than ten times that of oil palm, yet oil palm releases nearly ten times more oxygen into the atmosphere and absorbs nearly ten times more carbon dioxide (a major contributor to global warming).

The Brazilian government acknowledged the loss of 5,420 square miles of rainforest in just one year. This is an area more than twice the size as the entire state of Delaware! The good news is that the Brazilian Environment Ministry reported that the rate of Amazon destruction dropped 20 percent. Why the slowdown? You can thank the palm oil producers. Competition with palm oil has lowered the demand for soybean oil causing the soybean market to decline. With less of a demand for soybean oil, there is less incentive to clear the Amazon rainforest. The rising demand for palm oil (much of it as a replacement for hydrogenated soybean oil) has made a significant impact in slowing down the careless, yet legal, destruction of the Amazon.

The mandatory labeling law in the US that requires food manufacturers to list the trans fat content on their food labels has caused a decline in the demand for hydrogenated soybean oil. As a consequence, demand for palm oil has increased. In 2007, the first year after the law went into effect, the shift to palm oil saved 1,087 square miles of Amazon rainforest from being leveled for soybean cultivation.[4] Some people might look at this and say, but places like Malaysia (one of the world's biggest palm oil producers) also convert rainforest into farmland. However, in the past four years, even with the decline in demand for soybean oil, more Amazon rainforest in Brazil has been destroyed to make room for soybean cultivation than Malaysia has cleared in the past 100 years for palm oil production. Do the math. When you compare palm oil to soybean, and in fact to any other oil crop, palm oil is by far the most environmentally friendly. There is no comparison. Hopefully, as demand for palm oil increases, the demand for soybean oil will decrease, saving even more of the Amazon rainforest, and the earth as a whole, from needless destruction.

Has there been abuse in the palm oil industry? Yes. Some illegal operations have cut rainforests and displaced wildlife to plant palm plantations. But this is the exception, and very uncommon. Unfortunately, it is these rare abuses that get worldwide publicity and paint a misleading picture that this sort of thing is the norm. But what about the abuse that occurs with other crops? More rainforests and virgin land has been illegally and legally destroyed for the cultivation of soybeans, canola, and corn than has been converted to palm oil. Much of the land is cleared not only for soybeans, but for GE soybeans, canola, and corn, which wreak havoc on the environment, destroys the soil, kills wildlife, and harms human health. Do we hear anything about that?

Despite the massive destruction caused by the soybean industry, you never hear people crying out against the use of soybean oil. You don't see CSPI or Friends of the Earth attacking the soybean industry for destroying the environment. Why is that? Why are the environmental and consumer advocate groups mysteriously quiet about soy, yet violently active against the palm oil industry? The answer is power, greed, and misinformation. The seed oil industry is very rich and powerful. They know how to manipulate the media and these special interest groups and use them as unsuspecting puppets to spread their propaganda. They feed them lies, half-truths, and misconceptions in order to con them and the public.

If the seed oil industry wins the war against palm oil what would be the consequences? Without palm oil, the need for editable oils will be taken up by seed oil products—soybean, corn, canola, cottonseed, and others, the vast majority of which is GE. That means more deforestation of the Amazon, Argentina, Malaysia, Indonesia, and elsewhere to provide the land for seed oil cultivation. The Asian countries that were exporting palm oil will be forced to cut down the palm oil trees and convert the land to soy and other seed oil crops. They will have to do this to replace the lost revenue from palm oil to prevent a financial crisis for the country and its people. It will be either plant soy or starve. Since seed oils need 10 to 20 times as much land to produce the same amount of oil, vast areas of virgin tropical rainforest, as well as grasslands, and other land will be converted to biotech agriculture, growing GE crops and be sprayed heavily with disease-causing, environment-destroying pesticides. In addition, the land itself will be dug up and plowed, all native vegetation will be destroyed to make room for the new crops. Wildlife will be driven from their homes or killed, like never before. The soil will be altered by pesticides and synthetic fertilizers, changing the ecology of the soil microorganisms and the land forever. It would become an environmental nightmare! This would be the worse move we could make to protect the planet.

Prior to 2006, the year in which the new trans fat labeling laws went into effect, you never heard about all of the alleged environmental devastation caused by the palm oil industry. Prior to that time soybean oil was the most widely traded oil on the world market. Partially hydrogenated vegetable oils, margarine, or shortening were in the majority of our packaged foods. Business was booming for the seed oil industry. But as soon as these oils began to be replaced by palm oil, suddenly there was an outcry that the palm oil industry was destroying the planet. Where were these protestors prior to this time? Palm oil has been around for many decades. Why all of the sudden are these alleged environmental atrocities now front page news? If these abuses really were occurring, why were they not noted before 2006?

You can tell who is behind any scheme by following the money. Who stands to profit most from the downfall of the palm oil industry? The obvious benefactors are the powerful seed oil companies in North America and Europe who will rapidly fill the void left by the demise of palm oil; and, of course, Monsanto who sells GE seeds and chemicals. Who stands to lose? The hundreds of thousands of farm owners and laborers living in developing countries like Malaysia, Indonesia, Nigeria, Ghana, Kenya, and Colombia, who depend on palm oil for their livelihoods. The wildlife and environment will also suffer. And so will you and me as health-promoting palm oil is replaced by harmful GE seed oils in our foods.

If only the green organizations would wake up and recognize these facts and stop their blind persecution of palm oil. It is diabolically clever how the organizations and companies that pose the greatest threat to the planet are using green organizations as unwitting pawns to advance their agenda. How ironic it is that the efforts of these green groups to save the planet, could possibly be playing a major role in destroying it.

The campaign against palm oil is terribly deceitful and compelling. Pictures are used to evoke sympathy and outrage. It doesn't matter if the picture has nothing to do with palm oil. If it can be used as ammunition, it will. Nothing is more heart wrenching than seeing the abuse of an animal, such as the human-like orangutan. Any picture of an abused or injured orangutan is fair game to spread propaganda, as evidenced by the news story in the UK press about the orangutan that was allegedly confined in a cage all its life by heartless palm growers. However, it was discovered that the animal actually received medical treatment and was being transferred back into the wild. The picture of the caged animal had nothing to do with palm oil. The same is true with numerous other photos used to sway public opinion against the use of palm oil. People just assume that a graphic picture accompanying an alarming headline is actually associated with the text, they have no idea it is all just a clever marketing ploy.

A picture depicting a tropical rainforest being cut down is accompanied by a headline proclaiming that rainforests are being cleared at the rate of 300 football fields every hour, just in Indonesia alone. At such a ridiculous rate, all the forests in the country would be leveled in months. And the picture accompanying the headline, most likely is not associated with palm oil at all. There is no evidence to show an association. More likely, the land is being cleared for soybean cultivation, as far more rainforests are cleared for that purpose.

The campaign against palm oil isn't going away anytime soon. In the following months and years you will no doubt hear many graphic reports depicting how palm oil cultivation is destroying the earth, contributing to greenhouse gases, and driving animals into extinction. You will hear little or nothing about the destruction caused by the seed oils. The truth is that palm oil cultivation has only a minor impact on the environment. Most of the cultivation is done in a very environmentally friendly manner. So don't be fooled. The real danger is coming from the soybean and seed oil industries. It took us three decades to realize the harm the soybean industry caused to our health with the replacement of tropical oils with hydrogenated soybean oil. Let's not make another mistake with our environment.

Soybean Versus Oil Palm Cultivation

Soybean Cultivation

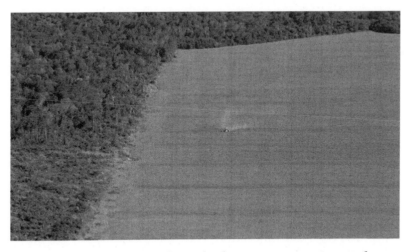

Brazilian rainforest is cleared of native vegetation and prepared for soybean cultivation.

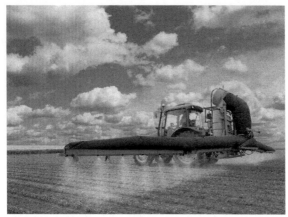

Soy seedlings being sprayed. Rainwater, native vegetation, and soil are poisoned by the repeated use of pesticides and the extensive cultivation.

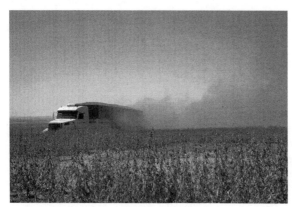

Harvesting and trucking of the mature soy.

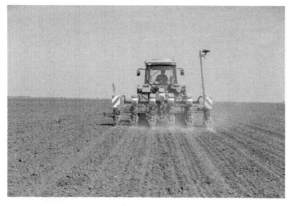

Plowing and reseeding the ground. The cycle begins all over and continues year after year. The land is void of native vegetation and wildlife.

Oil Palm Cultivation

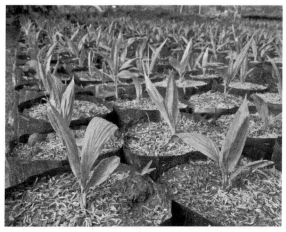

Oil palm seedlings are grown in nurseries before being planted in the field. Large scale plowing and soil cultivation is unnecessary leaving the soil ecology largely unchanged.

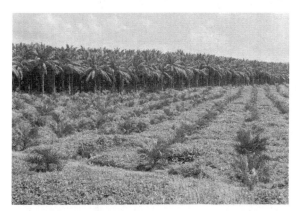

Oil palm farm with mixed young and mature oil palms (Malaysia). No GMO plants or herbicide sprays are used.

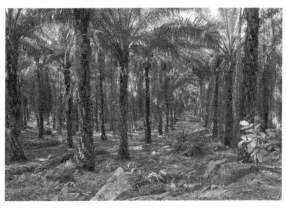

Mature oil palm plantations look much like tropical rainforests with native wildlife. Note the rich organic matter on the ground that provide natural fertilizer for the soil.

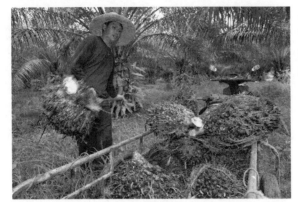

Palm fruit is harvested by hand not by tractors or machinery.

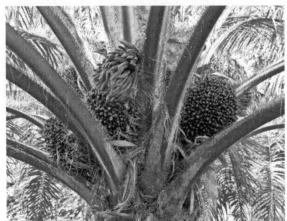

Oil palms produce fruit continually throughout the year and remain productive for 25 years or more. During this time the soil and wildlife remain largely undisturbed.

Soy

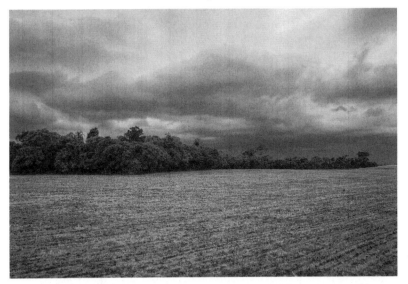

Soybean field in Mato Grosso Brazil (Amazon Basin).

Palm

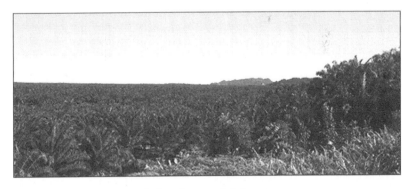

Oil palms in Malaysia.

Soy or palm, which one is more ecologically friendly? When given the truth, it doesn't take a genius to recognize the answer.

References

Chapter 2

1. Tomeo, A.C., et al. Antioxidant effects of tocotrienols in patients with hyperlipidemia and carotid stenosis. Lipids 1995;30:1179-1183.

2. Qureshi, A.A., et al. Response of Hypercholesterolemic subjects to administration of tocotrienols. *Lipids* 1995;30:1171-1177.

3. Tan, D.T.S., et al. Effect of a palm-oil-vitamin E concentrate on the serum and lipoprotein lipids in humans. *Am J Clin Nutr* 1991;53Suppl:1027S-1030S.

4. Theriault, A., et al Tocotrienol: a review of its therapeutic potential. *Clin Biochem* 1999;32:309-319.

5. Wood, R., et al. Effect of palm oil, margarine, butter and sunflower oil on the serum lipids and lipoproteins of normocholesterolemic middle-aged men. *J Nutr Bio Chem* 1993;4:286-297.

6. Esterhuyse, A.J., et al. Dietary red palm oil supplementation protects against the consequences of global ischemia in the isolated perfused rat heart. *Asia Pac J Clin Nutr* 2005;14:340-347.

7. Sron, B. Palm oil's track record. *Global Oil and Fats* 2005;2:24-25.

8. Yano, Y., et al. Induction of cytotoxicity in human lung adenocarcinoma cells by 6-0-carboxypropyl-alpha-tocotrienol, a redox-silent derivative of alpha-tocotrienol. *Int J Cancer* 2005;115:839-846.

9. Khanna, S. et al. Molecular basis of vitamin E action: tocotrienol modulates 12-lipoxygenase, a key moderator of glutamate-induced neurodegeneration. *J Biol Chem* 2003;278:43508-43515.

Chapter 4

1. Latham, JR, et al. Transformation-induced mutations in transgenic plants: analysis and biosafety implications. *Biotechnol Genet Eng Rev* 2006;23:209-237.

2. Bohn, T, et al. Compositional differences in soybeans on the market: glyphosate accumulates in Roundup Ready GM soybeans. *Food Chem* 2014;15:207-215.

3. Gasnier, C, et al. Glyphosate-based herbicides are toxic and endocrine distruptors in human cell lines. *Toxicology* 2009;262:184-191.

4. https://www.geneticliteracyproject.org/2014/03/05/controversial-iowa-farmer-howard-vlieger-makes-case-against-gmos/.

5. www.GMOjudycarman.org.

6. Carman, JA, et al. A long-term toxicology study on pigs fed a combined genetically modified (GM) soy and GM maize diet. *Journal of Organic System* 2013;8:38-54.

7. Seralini, G-E, et al. Long term toxicity of a roundup herbicide and a roundup-tolerant genetically modified maize. *Food and Chemical Toxicology* 2012;50:4221-4231.

Chapter 5
1. Samsel, A. and Seneff, S. Glyphosate's suppression of cytochrome P450 enzymes and amino acid biosynthesis by the gut microbiome: pathways to modern diseases. *Entropy* 2013;15:1416-1463.

2. Gasnier, C., et al. Glyphosate-based herbicides are toxic and endocrine disruptors in human cell lines. *Toxicology* 2009, 262, 184–191.

3. Kim, Y.H, et al. Mixtures of glyphosate and surfactant TN20 accelerate cell death via mitochondrial damage-induced apoptosis and necrosis. *Toxicol. In Vitro* 2013, 27, 191–197.

4. Paganelli, A, et al. glyphosate-based herbicides produce teratogenic effects on vertebrates by impairing retinoic acid signaling. *Chem Res Toxicol* 2010;23:1586-1595.

Chapter 6
1. Hunter, BT. How a PR campaign led to unhealthy diets. *Consumers' Research* 2003;86 (8).

2. http://www.freemalaysiatoday.com/category/opinion/2012/06/06/malaysian-palm-oil-and-eu-taxpayer-funding-campaigns/

3. Wallace, S. Last of the Amazon. *National Geographic* 2007;211:40-71.

4. Lehman, S. Brazil says Amazon deforestation is down. *USA Today* December, 7, 2007.

Index

The Palm Oil Miracle

Palm oil has been used as both a food and a medicine for thousands of years. it was prized by the pharaohs of ancient Egypt as a sacred food. Today palm oil is the most widely used oil in the world. In tropical Africa and Southeast Asia it is an integral part of a healthy diet just as olive oil is in the Mediterranean.

Palm oil possesses excellent cooking properties. It is more heat stable than other vegetable oils and imparts in foods and baked goods superior taste, texture, and quality.

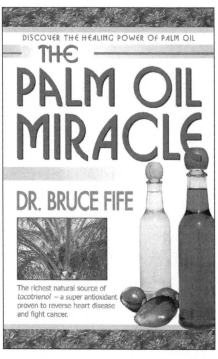

Palm oil is one of the world's healthiest oils. As a natural vegetable oil, it contains no trans fatty acids or cholesterol. It is currently being used by doctors and government agencies to treat specific illnesses and improve nutritional status. Recent medical studies have shown that palm oil, particularly virgin (red) palm oil, can protect against many common health problems. Some of the health benefits include:

To get your copy of *The Palm Oil Miracle* go to
www.piccadillybooks.com.

Some of the many properties of palm oil:

- Improves blood circulation
- Protects against heart disease
- Protects against cancer
- Boosts immunity
- Improves blood sugar control
- Improves nutrient absorption and vitamin and mineral status
- Aids in the prevention and treatment of malnutrition
- Supports healthy lung function
- Supports healthy liver function
- Helps strengthen bones and teeth
- Supports eye health
- Highest natural source of health promoting tocotrienols
- Helps protect against mental deterioration, including Alzheimer's disease
- Richest dietary source of vitamin E and beta-carotene

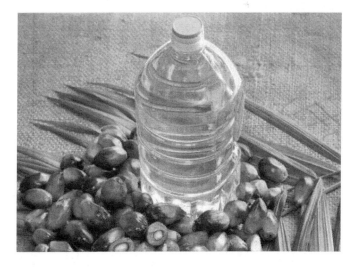

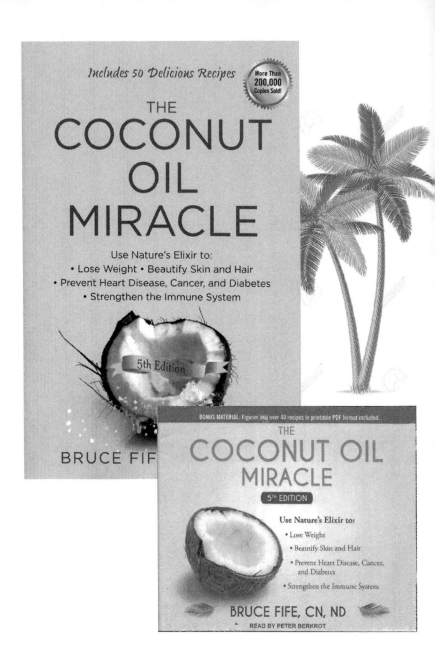

Visit Us on the Web

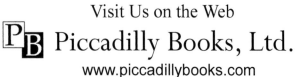 Piccadilly Books, Ltd.

www.piccadillybooks.com

35767959R00050

Printed in Great Britain
by Amazon